A Sociological Approach *to* Health Determinants

A Sociological Approach to Health Determinants investigates how 'the social' works in determining health and health inequity. Taking a global perspective, the book shines a light on how experiences of health, illness and health care are shaped by a variety of complex social dynamics.

Informed primarily by sociology, the book engages with the WHO's social determinants of health approach and draws on contributions from history, political economy and policy analysis to examine issues such as class, gender, ethnicity and indigeneity, and the impact they have on health.

A Sociological Approach to Health Determinants is a comprehensive resource that provides a new perspective on the influence of social structures on health, and how our understanding of the social can ensure improved health outcomes for people all over the globe.

Additional resources for instructors are available online at www.cambridge.edu.au/academic/socialdeterminants

Toni Schofield is Associate Professor (Honorary) at The University of Sydney.

A Sociological Approach

to Health Determinants

Toni Schofield

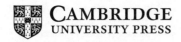

CAMBRIDGE
UNIVERSITY PRESS

CAMBRIDGE
UNIVERSITY PRESS

477 Williamstown Road, Port Melbourne, VIC 3207, Australia

Cambridge University Press is part of the University of Cambridge.

It furthers the University's mission by disseminating knowledge in the pursuit of education, learning and research at the highest international levels of excellence.

www.cambridge.org

Information on this title: www.cambridge.org/9781107689411

First published 2015

Cover designed by Zo Gay
Typeset by Aptara Corp.
Printed in China by C & C Offset Printing Co. Ltd.

A catalogue record for this publication is available from the British Library

A Cataloguing-in-Publication entry is available from the catalogue of the National Library of Australia at www.nla.gov.au

ISBN 978-1-107-68941-1 Paperback

Additional resources for this publication at www.cambridge.edu.au/academic/socialdeterminants

Every effort has been made in preparing this book to provide accurate and up-to-date information that is in accord with accepted standards and practice at the time of publication. Although case histories are drawn from actual cases, every effort has been made to disguise the identities of the individuals involved. Nevertheless, the authors, editors and publishers can make no warranties that the information contained herein is totally free from error, not least because clinical standards are constantly changing through research and regulation. The authors, editors and publishers therefore disclaim all liability for direct or consequential damages resulting from the use of material contained in this book. Readers are strongly advised to pay careful attention to information provided by the manufacturer of any drugs or equipment that they plan to use.

Foreword

'To good health!' we say when sharing a drink. Sadly, all too often that good health is not shared. Many people do not enjoy the conditions needed to live healthy lives.

Health authorities around the world now recognise the social determinants of health as a major concern. That is an important advance. Recognising a problem, however, and understanding it, are different things. And doing something effective about it is another matter again.

In this book Toni Schofield and her colleagues move us towards understanding and action. They give the facts about health and society, mapping the realities of class, gender, ethnicity, indigeneity, the state and health care. The facts are tough. There is grim evidence here about violence, abuse and exclusion; and about the less-dramatic, grinding effects of poverty and stress.

The book does much more. It takes us beyond describing the social dimensions of health to the 'causes of the causes' – the social *dynamics* of health. The chapters consider carefully the major structures of inequality in contemporary societies, explaining how they operate and how they have changed. They place health in the context of economic change, colonisation, migration and changing reproductive practices.

How do social inequalities get under the skin and become health effects? That's a key question, and in this book we see the multiple answers. They range from socially caused malnutrition, to social pathways of viral infection, to physical injury in the workplace, to genetic damage and environmental pollution. All are bound up in the operations of social power. All have an impact on bodies, but unequally so.

This book combines contemporary social analysis, a rich assembly of evidence about health in social contexts and illuminating vignettes of lives and situations. It is both accessible and intelligent. It has humour, detail and global sweep, inviting us to think about society and health where we live, and on a world scale.

The authors deal with issues that matter, and do not pull punches. They explore the ways in which business-friendly governments, bent on expanding the power of the market and opportunities for profit, may now be undermining past gains in community health. They explore the long-term effects of colonisation on Aboriginal peoples as well as the historic trauma. Without being pompous, this is a morally serious book.

There is vital information for health professionals and educators, here. The social determinants of health are now an established issue in health policy; and this book shows how practitioners can understand that issue.

It is also of wider interest. The issues discussed here are large contemporary questions of social justice and our collective well-being. Any citizen concerned with the state of our world can learn from this book, and learn things that matter.

Raewyn Connell
Professor Emerita
The University of Sydney
April 2014

Contents

Acknowledgements

Writing a book demands a lot of time in one's own company. This book was no different. Yet, such a project is also quintessentially social. In my case – and I suspect in most, if not all, cases – I relied on a small army of people to enable me to finish and deliver the final product. First were my co-authors in several of the book's chapters: Marco Berti, Michelle Donelly, John Gilroy and Christina Ho. Each brought a distinctive, scholarly and critical eye to the social determinants of health and the social–scientific sources we used to make sense of them. I am indebted to their contributions. I also benefited immeasurably from the research and editorial assistance provided by Bec O'Brien and my son, Eugene Schofield-Georgeson – both of whom insisted that all was not lost when I showed signs of losing the plot. In ensuring that the book's tables and figures would be as technically accomplished as they possibly could be, I also owe Peter Willey very considerable thanks. So, too, Patricia Corbett for her invaluable administrative help.

There were two key Cambridge University Press people whom I would also like to acknowledge for their expert contributions to this book: Nina Sharpe, who commissioned it and shepherded it to completion, and Renée Otmar, a consultant who provided rigorous editing and proofreading support.

As mentor extraordinaire for much of my intellectual life, Raewyn Connell paid me the great honour of reading most of the book when it was in draft form. As any experienced academic writer can attest, reading drafts of any kind of scholarship can be a 'challenge' in drumming up favourable comments. Raewyn, however, managed to do so, as her generous foreword shows. I am also grateful to other colleagues with whom I have worked over the past couple of years in teaching and researching. They did not necessarily make explicit contributions to the text but their intellectual collegiality and friendship have been critical in maintaining my engagement with the project of critical thinking, reading and writing. Johanna Adriaanse, Rebecca Brown, Fran Collyer, Susan Goff, Julie Hepworth, Maree Herrett, Dianna Kenny, Rose Leontini, Ron McCallum, Helen Meekosha, Cristiana Palmieri, Kerreen Reiger, Belinda Reeve, Stephanie Short and Deirdre Wicks all unwittingly engaged and helped me in assimilating many of the ideas I have tried to develop in this book.

Love and support, of course, were big players in this project. For these, I am indebted to my son and his partner, Jesse Adams-Stein, to my longstanding best friend, Sue Carroll, to my mother and sister (Alma and Kim), and to my endlessly patient and loving partner, John James.

1 The social determinants of health approach

Overview

● What are health inequities according to a social determinants of health (SDOH) approach?

● What causes health inequities and how can they be abolished using this approach?

● What are the limitations of the SDOH approach in addressing and redressing health inequities?

Nigeria, around 1970

Jonathan Iwegbu counted himself extraordinarily lucky. 'Happy survival!' meant so much more to him than a current fashion of greeting old friends in the first hazy days of peace... He had come out of the war with five inestimable blessings – his head, his wife Maria's head and the heads of three out of their four children. As a bonus he also had his old bicycle – a miracle too but naturally not to be compared to the safety of five human heads...

... [Jonathan] made the journey to Enugu and found another miracle waiting for him. It was unbelievable...This newest miracle was his little house in Ogui Overside...Only two houses away a huge concrete edifice some wealthy contractor had put up just before the war was a mountain of rubble. And here was Jonathan's little zinc house of no regrets built with mud blocks quite intact! Of course the doors and windows were missing and five sheets off the roof. But what was that? And anyhow he had returned to Enugu early enough to pick up bits of old zinc and wood and soggy sheets of cardboard lying around the neighbourhood before thousands more came out of their forest holes looking for the same thing. He got a destitute carpenter with one old hammer, a blunt plane and a few bent and rusty nails in his tool bag to turn this assortment of wood, paper and metal into door and window shutters for five Nigerian shillings...

His children picked mangoes near the military cemetery and sold them to soldiers' wives for a few pennies...and his wife started making breakfast *akara* balls* for neighbours in a hurry to start life again. With his family earnings he took his bicycle to the villages around and bought fresh palm-wine which he mixed generously...with the water which had recently started running again in the public tap down the road, and opened up a bar for soldiers and other lucky people with good money. (Achebe, 1985: 29–30)

*Fried patties or cakes made with black beans, onions and sometimes chilli.

As the extract from a short story by Nigerian author Chinua Achebe suggests, this story starts in sub-Saharan Africa, on the western side of the continent. Evoking a popular stereotype of the region, Achebe's story recounts an experience of civil war and precarious survival; in this case one that occurred between 1967 and 1970 in Nigeria. The players have changed since then, as have the triggers of the conflicts, but violence and civil disruption persist, as does the struggle by Nigerians to feed, clothe and house themselves. These kinds of struggles are not peculiar to Nigerians. They characterise the lives of millions of people in sub-Saharan Africa, particularly those experiencing recent bloody warfare and/or civil upheaval in Liberia, Sierra Leone, Mali, the Democratic Republic of the Congo and other countries in the region (Straus 2013). Although there is much talk about diversification of exports, intensive development of trade and removal of trade barriers as the answers to the struggles of nations in sub-Saharan Africa (World Bank 2012), there is considerable doubt about how successful such approaches would be in enhancing the lives of most sub-Saharan Africans (Cornelissen, Cheru and Shaw 2012).

As a region, sub-Saharan Africa has been a major exporter of resources, especially gold and other minerals from the western region, at least since the ninth century (Wolf 1982). The exportation of people as slaves from both the eastern and western regions of the continent is estimated to have begun around the same time. Less commonly acknowledged is the departure of people from East Africa who were not slaves, significantly pre-dating this trade – around 60 000 years ago (Stringer 2012). These were the first 'modern humans', or *homo sapiens* – the ancestors of all the planet's present inhabitants, including, of course, contemporary Africans (Stringer 2012). Estimated to be fewer than 1000, they walked out of the continent over 60 000 years ago and initially dispersed across Asia (Stringer 2012). We – their descendants – now number close to 7 billion and, while we share pretty much the same genetic make-up, our diversity has proliferated. We not only differ in physical appearance and language, but also in our histories, use of the physical environment and the myriad practices and technologies that comprise what we call 'a way of life'.

This diversity now commands considerable scientific interest from an army of researchers including anthropologists, archaeologists, geneticists, geographers, historians, philologists, sociologists and so on. Each specialises in particular aspects of this diversity. Two of the most significant specialities – and the focus of this book – is human health and health care, and how these are linked to the circumstances of people's lives and the ways in which they live.

By studying human health and health care, we can know with great certainty that the Nigerian experience of struggling to survive, for example, is accompanied by shortened lifespan, chronic illness and disability, and a loss of life in childbirth and infancy that is among the worst in the world (UNICEF 2013). We also know that as we move from Nigeria towards more northern latitudes and easterly across the globe to the United Kingdom, Scandinavia, Japan and Canada, for example, peoples' health could hardly be more different. Despite variations in language, history, geography and so on, these countries share a health bounty that sees the great majority reaching old age (over 65 years) (WHO 2013c) and generally supported with high-quality hospital and medical services. Well-nourished – in fact, excessively so in the United Kingdom and Canada, according to their governments' figures on the weight of their respective populations (WHO 2013e) – most, if not all of these northerners' encounters with hunger and pervasive mortality are typically confined to their consumption of electronic media.

Yet, dipping south from this easterly trajectory to the countries of South Asia, including India, it is evident that widespread immiseration, disease and premature death are not virtual realities. Like large swathes of the people in sub-Saharan Africa, literally hundreds of millions of Indians experience lives that are 'nasty, brutish and short' – and without access even to basic health services and medications. For many northerners, this experience is a cliché – life in the 'third world'. For the central character in a novel created by one of India's most celebrated authors (Adiga 2008), such a life is no cliché. As the satirical account (see box) of his childhood village home suggests, and as he comments frequently with respect to life in India, 'it's a f...ing joke!'

India, the early 2000s

Laxmangarh is your typical Indian village paradise, adequately supplied with electricity, running water, and working telephones; and...the children...raised on a nutritious diet of meat, eggs, vegetables, and lentils, will be found, when examined with tape measure and scales, to match up to the minimum height and weight standards set by the United Nations and other organizations whose treaties our prime minister has signed and whose forums he so regularly and pompously attends.

Ha!
Electricity poles – defunct.
Water tap – broken.

Children – too lean and short for their age, and with over-sized heads from which vivid eyes shine, like the guilty conscience of the government of India.

Yes, a typical Indian village paradise...
Down the middle of the main road, families of pigs are sniffing through sewage... Past the hogs and roosters, you'll get to my house – if it still exists.
At the doorway to my house, you'll see the most important member of my family.

The water buffalo
She was the fattest thing in our family; this was true in every house in the village. All day long, the women fed her... feeding her was the main thing in their lives... If she gave enough milk, the women could sell some of it, and there might be a little more money at the end of the day. (Adiga 2008: 19–20)

Travelling east from India, crossing the Equator and moving south, we reach Australia – the home of the oldest direct descendants of those who walked out of Africa all those years ago. Now called 'Indigenous or Aboriginal Australians', they cohabit with predominantly European people whose forbears first arrived from England in the late 18th century by boat. Entering the island continent from the city of Darwin in the Northern Territory (NT), we see that the signs of affluence evident in the countries of the northern latitudes mentioned previously are everywhere here as well. Well-maintained public amenities to support the health and well-being of its people, most of whom are expected to live well into their 70s and 80s (WHO 2013c), are one such feature. Especially popular among these is the iconic public swimming pool. A well-known Australian children's author, Libby Gleeson (1993), illustrates through the eyes of one of her teenaged protagonists the centrality of the public swimming pool in the lives of many Australians, especially young people, and the taken-for-granted physical and other, less tangible but pleasurable, health benefits they derive from it. Doing laps, for instance, not only serves as a vigorous form of physical activity but allows him time for self-reflection. As he comments, '[I get to] think about all sorts of stuff, arguments I've had, conversations and what I should've said. Other times it's like the water washes your brain out' (Gleeson 1993: 153). And when 'other kids are there... we always muck around and have a good time' (Gleeson 1993: 152).

Yet, a tour of Darwin's public pools and the city's sprawling precincts reveals that the reassuring public amenity and tropical opulence encountered upon arrival are not the complete picture, especially with respect to the oldest direct descendants of homo sapiens from Africa. Though they number around 10 per cent of the city's population (Australian Bureau of Statistics (ABS) 2011), there are barely any Indigenous Australians at the pools. And they are not found taking a dip in Darwin's crocodile-infested beaches and streams, either. There are, however, large concentrations of Indigenous people living in makeshift camps and settlements in and around the city that evoke the poverty and squalor of Adiga's Indian villages. The health calculations of the Australian Institute of Health and Welfare (AIHW 2013c) suggest, in fact, that many Indigenous Australians across the country – especially those comprising about a third of the population in the NT (ABS 2006) – share similar sorts of health fortunes to those of the people encountered in Nigeria and India.

Health diversity: The WHO and the CSDH

Moving further east and north again to New York City, the most populous city in North America, we encounter the glass-and-steel headquarters of some of the world's largest international 'think tanks' and other organisations conducting research and providing information, advice, guidance and strategy on health and health care issues around the world. One of the most powerful of these is the United Nations (UN), and though it does not focus explicitly on health, the decisions and policies it produces have major effects on health internationally. The World Bank, not far from New York, in Washington DC, also plays a major role in producing policy and advice, and financing health interventions, discussed in more detail in Chapters 7 and 8. It is the World Health Organization (WHO), first established under the auspices of the UN in 1946, however, that exercises the greatest influence internationally in how the world's health issues are or should be understood, and how they should be addressed by national governments (Schofield 2007: 107–8). Further east and across the Atlantic Ocean to continental Europe, the WHO's headquarters are located in Geneva, Switzerland. Supported by regional offices throughout the world and a vast bureaucracy, the WHO has virtually no funds to finance the implementation of its proposals and no power to force governments to do so. It exercises influence largely because of its authority as a world leader in the scientific investigation and reporting of world health patterns and trends, and through taking the lead in coordinating and strategically planning 'global health' (Brown, Cueto and Fee 2006: 263).

So, what sense does the WHO make of the health diversity we have seen on our brief international tour? Communicating to the global public primarily through the worldwide web, the WHO's website showcases innumerable reports and publications. Among these, the one that engages most explicitly and comprehensively with health diversity on a global basis is *Closing the Gap in a Generation* (Commission on the Social Determinants of Health (CSDH) 2008). Almost 250 pages long, with lots of tables, graphs and charts, the report makes clear that, by contrast with much of human diversity, health diversity is no cause for celebration. In fact, according to the experts who researched, wrote and produced the report for the WHO, health differences of the kind we have seen are 'health inequities' – or unfair and unjust health differences (CSDH 2008: 1) – that have to be eliminated because they 'are killing people on a grand scale' (CSDH 2008: 248).

The CSDH has an unambiguous story to tell about global health inequities and how they can and should be abolished. At its heart is the idea of the 'social determinants of health'. The following excerpt from the *Closing the Gap* report introduces us to this idea from the WHO's perspective:

> The Commission takes a holistic view of social determinants of health. The poor health of the poor, the social gradient in health within countries, and the marked health inequities between countries are caused by the unequal distribution of power, income, goods, and services, globally and nationally, the consequent unfairness in the immediate, visible circumstances of peoples' lives – their access to health care, schools, and education, their conditions of work and leisure, their homes, communities, towns, or cities – and their chances of leading a flourishing life. This unequal distribution of health-damaging experiences is not in any sense a 'natural' phenomenon but is the result of a toxic combination of poor social policies and programmes, unfair economic arrangements, and bad politics. Together, the structural determinants and conditions of daily life constitute the social determinants of health and are responsible for a major part of health inequities between and within countries...
>
> And of course climate change has profound implications for . . . how it affects the way of life and health of individuals and the planet. We need to bring the two agendas of health equity and climate change together. (CSDH 2008: 1)

Even a cursory reading suggests that the social determinants of health are complex. The phrase, 'the social gradient in health' and the sentence, 'structural determinants and conditions of daily life constitute the social determinants of health', for instance, are unlikely to feature regularly, if at all, in most people's reading material and communications. Clarifying what the CSDH means by 'health' is a good start because it is central to the whole story, but there is no explicit definition or statement of what health is in the *Closing the Gap* report.

Yet, it is possible to identify what the report means by 'health' by analysing how it writes about – or represents – the topic.

'Health' and the WHO

The WHO has an official definition of health that was formulated in 1946 and has remained unamended since 1948. It proclaims that 'health is a state of complete physical, mental and social well-being and not merely the absence of disease or infirmity' (WHO 1948). A problem with this definition is that it represents health as a kind of transcendental experience, like heaven or nirvana. Not surprisingly, some have criticised it as unrealistic and utopian (Dubos 1960) – more like a definition of a spiritual state. It is certainly difficult to identify and measure. For the *Closing the Gap* report, by contrast, measurement is critical to how health is understood. The report presents itself first and foremost as a manifesto for action (CSDH 2008: 2) – global, national and local. In doing so, it stresses that the effectiveness or otherwise of its proposed actions need to be measured and assessed (CSDH 2008:2). Its actions, of course, are directed towards reducing and eliminating inequities in health, and the significance of measurement for the approach of the CSDH directly shapes its understanding of health. The measurement of health is a field of research developed by epidemiologists, who measure *health outcomes* or conditions related to death, illness, disease, injury, disability and expectation of years of life. The *Closing the Gap* (CSDH 2008: 182) report lists the following as health outcomes: 'mortality (all cause, cause specific, age specific); early childhood development; mental health; morbidity and disability; self-assessed physical and mental health; and cause-specific outcomes (mainly injuries).' Epidemiological terms for health outcomes are *technical,* as the following examples show.

Life expectancy is the average number of years an individual of a given age is expected to live if current mortality rates continue to apply on existing age-specific death rates (1).

Mortality rate is an estimate of the portion of a population that dies during a given time period (2).

All-cause mortality rate expresses the incidence of death from all causes in a population during a given time period (2).

Cause-specific mortality rate expresses the incidence of death from a specific cause in a population during a given time period (2).

Age-specific mortality rate expresses the incidence of death for a specific age group in a population during a given time period (2).

Morbidity refers to any departure, subjective or objective, from a state of physiological or psychological well-being (2).

(1) Last 2001
(2) Hennekens and Buring 1987

In measuring such outcomes, epidemiologists use statistical methods to calculate prevalence (total number) and incidence (number per 1000) among *populations*. They talk about *rates* of health outcomes such as the rate of maternal mortality, infant mortality, deaths from specific causes such as cardiovascular disease (CVD), deaths of adults between the ages of 18 and 65 years, and so on. In calculating the maternal mortality rate, for example, epidemiologists measure the number of women who die in pregnancy and childbirth as a proportion of a specific population of women who are pregnant or participate in childbirth, usually in any given year. In relation to morbidity, epidemiologists focus mainly on measuring disease conditions, both acute and chronic. To determine the rate of specific disease conditions such as cancer, CVD and HIV/AIDS, for example, they may measure the proportion of a particular population diagnosed with these conditions. Measures demonstrating a high prevalence or incidence of, say, mortality, morbidity or disability, generally indicate poor health, while low rates

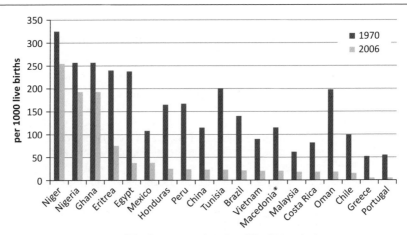

*The former Yugoslavic Republic of Macedonia

FIGURE 1.1

Under-5 mortality rates per 1000 live births, selected countries, 1970 and 2006
Source: Adapted from the original in CSDH 2008: 32.

indicate the opposite. Figure 1.1 is an example of the incidence of under-five year old deaths in a selection of 19 countries between 1970 and 2006 – an example of age-specific mortality.

The graph in Figure 1.1 shows the number of children under the age of five years who died as a proportion of 1000 live births by country in both 1970 and 2006. The countries shown are a selection only. The highest rate of under-five mortality among the 19 countries represented occurred in Niger, with more than 325 deaths per 1000 live births recorded in 1970 and a little over 250 recorded in 2006. The lowest rate, by contrast, occurred in Greece, with slightly more than 50 deaths recorded among under-five year old children for every 1000 live births in 1970 and approximately two for every 1000 live births in 2006. This graph permits comparisons, such as the rate of decline in the under-five mortality rate within and between selected countries for the period 1970–2006. Clearly, all countries disclosed a decline in the under-five death rate, but the greatest rate of decline was in Oman, judging by the height of the columns for 1970 and 2006. The country with the least or slowest rate of decline was Niger, but Nigeria and Ghana (all sub-Saharan African nations) also revealed rates of under-five mortality in 2006 that showed a markedly lower reduction since 1970 when compared with the other countries in the selection. On the basis of this one measure, it is evident that of the children under age five who are living in the selected 19 countries, those most likely to die are born in sub-Saharan Africa. Such a measure suggests that by comparison with their non sub-Saharan counterparts they are markedly less 'healthy'. This brings us to a further feature of the CSDH's understanding of health.

As the preceding has illustrated, epidemiologists are primarily concerned with the health of *populations* rather than *peoples*. A population is a statistical fabrication in the sense that the quantitative thinking and methods used to identify it actually create it or bring it into being (Schofield 2004, Rowse 2009). The first step in this process is to establish a boundary or marker of closure of the units to be included; the second step is to count the units. A fairly straightforward example is a national population. Here, the boundary is largely already drawn by agreement between and among nation states so that statisticians do not have to invent it. However, there are other factors that complicate the process, such as the residential and citizenship'status' of the units – or people – to be included. These operate as criteria that statisticians need to use in determining the boundaries of what they count in producing a population. A people, by contrast, is mainly but not exclusively used in regard to 'ethnic minorities' and those who are Indigenous to a particular region or country, such as the Indigenous peoples of Australia, North America and so on – a subject discussed further in the following chapter. It is a qualitative 'construction' that also involves the establishment of boundaries or distinctions, but the process is not undertaken by scientists such as statisticians or epidemiologists. These boundaries are drawn subjectively by a specific group of people who identify themselves as distinct from others, usually on the basis of their shared histories, ways of life, values and interests (Rowse 2009). As a result, they and their health are much more difficult for statisticians to measure than populations and their health, an issue explored further in Chapter 6.

In measuring health outcomes of populations, epidemiologists are usually interested in identifying *patterns*. As for many in the social sciences, they require a combination of measures to confidently identify the presence of a trend or pattern in human health. As we have seen above, the rate of under-five mortality per 1000 live births in 19 selected countries, for example, suggests that children under five years of age in sub-Saharan African countries are significantly less healthy than their counterparts in other parts of the world. Determining whether this illustrates a broader trend of significantly worse health in this region than other parts of the world requires the combination of a number of health outcome measures of a variety of population 'strata', of which children under age five is only one.

Health inequality and inequity

What should be evident by now is that epidemiological understandings of health, as defined by the WHO, for instance, are quantitative but they are used to make value judgements about whether human health is better or worse within and between populations. These judgements are based on measurable disparities or inequalities in health outcomes. Yet, the WHO's *Closing the Gap* report and its plans for action are not only concerned with health disparities but also with health inequities and their elimination. Is there a difference between health inequality and inequity? According to the WHO and the international community that is concerned with global health in an official capacity – comprised predominantly of researchers, policy makers and practitioners with expertise in what is called 'public health' – there is. Health inequalities of the kind illustrated in Figure 1.1 do not simply reflect magnitudes of difference in numbers of deaths. From a public health perspective, they reveal inequities because the observable, measurable inequalities are considered to be *avoidable* (CSDH 2008: 29). How are they avoidable? Public health experts agree that health inequities correlate strongly with, or are matched by, a combination of *social inequalities* (WHO 1990). These social inequalities are identified by a range of measures that apply to populations within countries, such as socio-economic status (usually comprised of a combination of measures, such as education, income, occupation and employment status), and between countries such as low, middle and high income. All of the members of the Organization for Economic Co-operation and Development (OECD), such as the United States, Japan, continental Europe, the United Kingdom, Australia and Canada, are high-income countries, as are several countries in the Persian Gulf, including Bahrain, Kuwait, Qatar, Saudi Arabia and the United Arab Emirates (WHO 2009a). Most of the countries in sub-Saharan Africa, by contrast, are low income. The remainder of the world's regions, accounting for most of the global population and including China, India, Indonesia, the states of the former Soviet Union and the countries of South America rank as low to middle-income countries (WHO 2009a). A further measure used to identify social inequalities both within and between countries is household wealth (see, for example, CSDH 2008: 31).

The *Closing the Gap* report provides numerous examples of health inequities, including:

> The prevalence of long-term disabilities among European men 80+ years is 58.8% among the lower educated versus 40.2% among the higher educated.

> An estimated 17.5 million people died from CVDs in 2005, representing 30% of all global deaths. Over 80% of CVD deaths occur in low- and middle-income countries.

> The lifetime risk of maternal death is one in eight in Afghanistan [a low-income country]; it is 1 in 17,400 in Sweden [a high-income country]. (CSDH 2008: 30)

Health inequities and social determinants

Where there are strong correlations or matches between health inequalities and social inequalities, epidemiologists and other public health experts (such as the members of the CSDH) propose the following. First, that the 'social factor' represented by the measure of social inequality – such as education, income, occupation or employment status (that is, employed, unemployed, self-employed, employer) – plays a *determining* role in the health outcome with which it is correlated. A social determinant of health, then, is basically a social factor characterised by measurable disparities (high, medium and low, for instance) that corresponds with inequalities in a particular health outcome (as indicated by lower and higher rates). It is in this sense that the *Closing the Gap* report proposes that health inequities are socially determined. Significantly, if a social factor is identified as determining of a health inequity then it is, by definition, unacceptable (CSDH 2008).

What is unacceptable about it derives from a further and fundamental feature of the WHO's understanding of health. When the WHO was established and proclaimed its definition of health, as previously mentioned, it also declared health a *universal human right*: 'The enjoyment of the highest attainable standard of health is one of the fundamental rights of every human being without distinction of race, religion, political belief, economic or social condition' (WHO 1948). As this declaration suggests, health cannot be contingent on any form of *social difference* or *distinction* because it is internationally recognised as an entitlement of each and every individual. This now prevailing understanding of health is a predominantly 'modern' construction, since at its heart is the idea that *individuals* matter. They matter in the sense that they are all of the same intrinsic worth or value, at the same time as being individually unique or irreplaceable. This idea, and its application to human health and health care, is pursued more extensively in the next chapter. What is important to emphasise here is that while the *Closing the Gap* report focuses on health inequities and their social determinants, the rationale for their elimination arises from a commitment to fairness and justice for all individuals. As the report comments, '… if the infant mortality rate in Iceland … were applied to the whole world, only two babies would die in every 1000 born alive' (CSDH 2008: 29).

The social determinants of health action plan

The social determinants of health approach as espoused by the WHO provides an understanding of health inequities that is committed to their elimination and an action plan for doing so. The plan's target comprises social inequality, specifically those inequalities associated with daily living conditions in which people 'are born, grow, live, work and age', and what is represented as the 'drivers of those conditions', namely the 'inequitable distribution of power, money and resources' (CSDH 2008: 2). The former are targeted because they are understood as the immediate causes of health inequalities, while the latter are the upstream causes – the 'causes of the causes'. The actions proposed to address and eliminate the causes mainly involve public policies and legislation – globally, nationally and locally – and changes in the ways that governments and corporations conduct their business, particularly in relation to facilitating greater 'bottom-up' participation. Here, the thinking is that enhanced 'inclusion' of the great diversity of people in the decision-making of these powerful organisations will promote increased opportunities for them to 'voice' their concerns and interests, and bring about change towards greater equality, an issue taken up in the following chapter.

There is no doubt, then, that according to the social determinants approach, 'social factors' that create massive inequalities in people's everyday lives lie at the heart of health inequities within and between countries. What is not so clear, and remains largely unanswered, is the question of what exactly produces the 'causes of the causes' and how 'causation' operates. How do inequities in 'power, money and resources' produce social inequalities, and how does the relationship between social inequalities and health outcomes actually work? The social determinants of health approach amply demonstrates consistent and robust correlations between social factors and health outcomes but it leaves largely unexplained why such associations exist in the first place and how they work. Why is such explanation important or relevant? As the *Closing the Gap* report itself emphasises, our knowledge and understanding of health inequities and their relationship to 'social determinants' are critical in informing and shaping effective interventions for change. As the history of medicine has demonstrated, knowledge and understanding of how the body and disease work have been crucial for producing many effective cures and relief of pain and suffering. Such knowledge and understanding provide a basis for action that avoids the pitfalls of trial-and-error approaches, whereby actions observed to be effective in a limited range of circumstances are adopted but the reasons for their efficacy are not understood. In the absence of knowledge that facilitates understanding of how things work – the principles and dynamics involved – it is difficult to identify the full range of possibilities for effective action. Identifying these principles and dynamics is intrinsic to scientific investigation and explanation.

The following chapters set out to address the questions raised above, providing a framework for understanding the relationship between health and 'the social' that moves beyond statistical correlations between health outcomes and social factors or indicators. In doing so, the book draws on a variety of knowledges, but the main one is *sociology*. The overarching purpose of this enterprise is to explore and explain what the social is and how it works, not simply in relation to the production and distribution of good and bad health both within and between countries. Its other main focus is the process by which the social 'gets under the skin' of individuals, producing the astonishing health disparities in people's daily experiences as embodied human beings. For some, as the following chapters will show, this experience is miserable and painful, seriously contracting the possibilities for participation in life, while for others it is pleasurable and energising, affording opportunities for participation that yield generous rewards. Like those of its public health counterparts, the account developed in this book does not adopt a disinterested or impartial stance towards health disparities. As the literary excerpts outlined at the beginning of this chapter suggest, what is at stake is far too real and confronting to pretend that such an approach is possible.

Conclusions

The world's population now numbers around 7 billion and, while we share much the same genetic make-up, peoples' health varies enormously across the globe. The health differences between high-income and low-to-middle-income countries, especially those of sub-Saharan Africa and South Asia, are actually 'health inequities' – or unfair and unjust health differences that have to be eliminated because they 'are killing people on a grand scale' (CSDH 2008).

According to the WHO, the unequal distribution of health-damaging experiences is not the outcome of natural differences but, rather, 'structural determinants and conditions of daily life' that comprise what they call the social determinants of health (CSDH 2008). Health inequities are evident in differential rates of health outcomes both within and between countries. These measures usually refer to patterns of health among specific populations and are related to a specific social factor such as income, wealth, education, occupation and so on. From this perspective, a social determinant of health is a social factor characterised by measurable disparities that corresponds with inequalities in a particular health outcome. A social factor identified as a determinant of health inequity is by definition unacceptable. This is because health is a universal human right that is not contingent on social difference or distinction.

The CSDH (2008) provides an action plan that is dedicated to eliminating health inequities by targeting the daily living conditions in which people 'are born, grow, live, work and age', and the 'drivers of those conditions', namely the 'inequitable distribution of power, money and resources'. The social determinants of health approach amply demonstrates consistent and robust correlations between social factors and health outcomes but it leaves largely unexplained why such associations exist in the first place and how they work. Such an approach is important because, as the WHO itself emphasises, our knowledge and understanding of health inequities and their relationship to 'social determinants' are critical in informing and shaping effective interventions for change.

There is a need, then, for a framework for understanding the relationship between health and 'the social' that moves beyond statistical correlations between health outcomes and social indicators. The following chapters identify and describe major health disparities within and between countries, drawing on significant epidemiological databases. However, the focuses of analysis and discussion are the social dynamics involved in generating social inequalities and *how they work* in producing the astonishing health disparities that prevail nationally and globally.

Questions for discussion

1   Which regions of the world have the most damaging health experiences? On what basis can we distinguish national or regional health profiles, and the differences between them? (See also the companion website to this text.)
2   How does the WHO's Commission on the Social Determinants of Health characterise health inequities, and why has it formulated a global plan to eliminate them?
3   How does the WHO's 1948 definition of health differ from the working definitions of health in the WHO's *Closing the Gap* report?
4   What does Figure 1.1 tell us about the health of the world's children under the age of five? To what extent does the picture of health suggested by this graph remain indicative of the general trend of young children's health throughout the world? (See companion website.)
5   What is the difference between 'peoples' and 'populations' in relation to health?
6   How does a social determinants of health approach represent the social in its identification of the social determinants of health? What are the limitations of this representation?

2 Understanding the social INTRODUCING SOCIOLOGY

Overview

- What does it mean to say that the individual is a 'modern' invention?

- In what ways were modernist ideas about the individual central to the development of 18th and 19th-century European thinking about the social?

- What is 'social structure' and what contribution does it make to understanding human being and action?

The Atlantic Ocean, somewhere between West Africa and South Carolina, 1756

The contractions began rolling hard and long and often, and I left it to Fanta (a slave woman) to decide when to push...

She pushed for a long time, and then she lay back and rested... 'Now,' Fanta said. She pushed three more times. I saw hairs on a head starting to part her, but the baby wouldn't come yet. She pushed once more, and the head came all the way out, blue and purplish and light coloured and specked with bits of whiteness and blood. Fanta pushed again, and out came the shoulders. The rest slid out quickly... I... slice[d] the cord, then I wrapped the baby and gave him to Fanta. The baby cried, and Fanta let it howl good and long before allowing it to root for her nipple. She was not a proud mother, but an angry one. I tried to settle Fanta comfortably on the bed, but she pushed me away. (Hill 2007: 86–7)

A few steps to my left, I saw Fanta crouching. At first, I thought she was injured or exhausted from the birth. She was doubled over, and the baby was wriggling on a cloth beside her. As I watched, Fanta reached inside her wrap. I heard the baby give a little cry. I saw his heels kicking. Fanta brought out the knife from the medicine man's room, placed a hand over the baby's face and jerked up his chin. She dug the tip of the knife into the baby's neck and ripped his throat open. Then she pulled the blue cloth over him, stood and heaved him overboard. (Hill 2007: 90)

This chapter starts in the 18th century and again in Africa. In this case, however, it is on the east coast of the continent and involves Africans' early encounters on a mass scale with Europeans. These Africans were captured – usually by tribal rulers engaged in hostilities against other tribes – and bartered to European companies and merchants mainly from Britain, France, Portugal and Holland (Hancock 1995: 214) – who in turn exported them by ship to be sold to work on plantations and farms in the West Indies and the British colonies in North America. This 18th-century, trans-Atlantic wave of slaves – the largest recorded since the start of European trade in Africa in the late 15th century (Adi 2012) – originated in the coastal and hinterland regions of Africa's west and was dominated by government and private merchants from Britain. Leaving ports such as Liverpool and Bristol, the British merchants loaded their ships to capacity with cloth and clothing, arms, metalware (pots, pans, cutlery, nails and locks, for example), foodstuffs (mainly tobacco and sugar), jewellery and miscellaneous goods to be unloaded and exchanged in west African harbours for their human cargo (Hancock 1995: 189–90). By the early 1800s, the industry began to decline and 'slaving' was gradually abolished. In Britain, the greatest European beneficiary of the trade, this occurred by an Act of parliament in 1833 (Blackburn 2012, Geggus 2012). It was not until the late 19th century, however, that the slave trade was formally outlawed in most parts of the world, by which time almost 12 million Africans had been forceably exported across the Atlantic (Lovejoy 1989: 368) to work in servitude.

As Canada's Lawrence Hill (2007) recounted above through the eyes of his central character, Aminata – a pubescent young woman captured by slave traders in 1756 – the trans-Atlantic slave trade of the 1700s was unspeakably violent and barbaric. Such an experience appears to have been associated with a kind of paradox. On the one hand, slaves were valued by traders and owners for their human-ness, particularly their human capacities to communicate with, and work as prescribed by, their owners, even reproducing for them. On the other hand, the realisation of this value depended on a refusal by slave owners and traders to recognise the *personhood* of the human beings they captured by selling and buying them, like any other market commodity. In other words, a slave was a human being who became the legal *private property* of another or others and, as such, able to be bought and sold at the absolute discretion of an owner. The fate of Fanta and her newborn baby on board a slave ship from West Africa to Carolina in the United States in 1756 illustrates the experience of this human effacement as well as resistance to it. Born to a slave mother, a baby automatically became the property of the mother's owner. Such was Fanta's rage and resistance to this prospect she killed her own newborn.

Slavery, of course, prevailed not only between Europeans and Africans, and not only in the 18th century, as mentioned in the previous chapter. In fact, though slavery is illegal everywhere today, some argue that it continues on a global basis with an estimated 27 million people – predominantly women and children – forced into servitude through human trafficking (Bales 2012). Yet, the trans-Atlantic slaving that occurred in the 18th century is especially significant not only because of its unprecedented scale. The industry was grown and managed by exporting and importing countries that were simultaneously cultivating a 'personage' that heralded its very demise. Such a character still exercises considerable power today – possibly more now than it ever has. This is 'the individual' (Williams 1976: 133–6). Though it may seem paradoxical, understanding the social and how it works in relation to health begins with discussion of this major historical actor. We turn now to the late 20th century and one of the most famous speeches ever made by a prime minister of the country in which the individual was passionately nurtured as an infant from the 17th century (Hill 1972). The country is Britain and the prime minister is the first woman to have held the office in that country – Dame Margaret Thatcher.

The individual and society

> There is no such thing [as society]! There are individual men and women and...families. [N]o government can do anything except through... [these individuals]. It is our duty to look after ourselves and...our neighbour [because] life is a reciprocal business...[So] there is no such thing as an entitlement unless someone has first met an obligation. (Thatcher 1987)

As Dame Thatcher's comments suggest, there is a lot riding on *her* individual. It basically all starts and ends with him or her. There is the family, of course, but in the end there is stand-alone 'you' and stand-alone 'me' – all of us individuals who have no choice but to get on with looking after ourselves independently of each other, save for some help for 'our neighbour'. Yet, Dame Thatcher's individual is not one entirely of her own invention. It is closely related to the concept of the individual that was generated in the 1600s mainly in Europe, but also in the 1700s in the United States, as part of a movement about the nature of human 'being and action' called the *Enlightenment* (Williams 1999, Lukes 1973). By contrast with Dame Thatcher's individual, however, the Enlightenment concept of the individual is rather more complicated; this approach is so important to an understanding of the concept that we need to take some time here to explain it a little further: but first, a clarification.

To say that 'the individual' did not appear and develop until the 17th century in Europe is not to suggest that individual people did not exist until then. Clearly, they did and their descendants – namely, us – also exist as real, flesh-and-blood individuals. Yet, how we understand ourselves as individual human beings has changed over time – and place. It is obvious that our ideas and thinking about ourselves as individuals are foundational to how we act and what we become over time. So the kinds of ideas and thinking we adopt in the process – what sociologists call *symbolisation* or *representation* – are critical (see Chapter 3). Not that being and becoming an individual only involves such a process – far from it, particularly as current research on infant development shows (see Kenny 2013, for a comprehensive review). We are and become individuals through our *bodies*, including how we think and understand the world (Gilman 2000, 2010). It cannot happen by any other means. As mentioned above, however, it was Enlightenment thinking about people as individuals that dramatically shaped the ways in which large swathes of the world's peoples conceive of themselves and participate in their lives. This effect has been most pronounced among peoples of European (including British) origins, but Enlightenment ideas have spread among non-European peoples across the globe as Europeans became dispersed and established themselves in the Americas, Africa, Asia and the South Pacific. This process of colonisation (see Chapters 5 and 6) usually involved the ruthless supplanting of the inhabitants' ways of life with those of Europeans, and the disparagement and erasure of Indigenous ways of thinking about human being and action (Smith 2012). In many cases, however, Indigenous peoples resisted and struggled to assert their pre-colonised thinking, or to synthesise it with Enlightenment ideas as they did in parts of the colonised world (Connell 2007).

One of the outstanding features of Enlightenment thinking was that people are individuals who should be distinguished and valued as *persons*, each of whom 'exists as an end in himself [sic], not merely as a means [for use by others]...' (Kant 1785, cited in Lukes 1973: 49). This Kantian understanding – so-named in honour of its author, the German philosopher Immanuel Kant – asserted the *innate dignity* and worth of each and every individual. All individuals should have the same value as each other – or be *equal* – but also be simultaneously valued for their individual specificity or distinctiveness: *the same but different*. Second, individual persons should be *autonomous*, or self-directed in the sense that they should be free and able to think for themselves (Lukes 1973: 52–8). They should adopt reason to determine what they believe and how they should act, not blindly obey prevailing orthodoxies. Third, individuals should have *privacy* – an area of existence of no concern to others (Lukes 1973: 59–66), including 'the public' and 'the state' (see Chapter 7). The private sphere is the place in which individuals can and should do whatever they like, especially with respect to family relationships and property, as long as this 'causes no harm to others'. Fourth and finally, individuals should engage in *self-development* because personhood demands active and wide-ranging *participation* in life in order to facilitate the 'flowering' of talents and abilities from which all can benefit (Lukes 1973: 67–72).

These ideals and values about individuals emerged as part of a radical break with the thinking and beliefs espoused by religions and monarchies that dominated and shaped what is often described as *pre-modernity* (Berman 1988, Giddens 1991) in Europe – a time and a place characterised by medieval cosmologies that placed god at the centre of the universe and as the creator of everything, including human destiny. Human beings basically existed to do what god had ordained – at least as 'his' representatives on earth (the churches and the monarchies) interpreted it. As a key element of the departure from this way of thinking, the Enlightenment simultaneously played a groundbreaking role in bringing *modernity* (Berman 1988, Geras and Wokler 2000) into being. One of the most significant ways in which the 'early moderns', such as the hundreds of 18th-century French *philosophes* (most notably Diderot, Voltaire, Rousseau and Montesquieu), defined and understood individuals was as stand-alone human beings – like those in Dame Thatcher's speech. '(E)ach individual . . . is by himself [sic] a complete and solitary whole . . .' according to one of France's most-renowned early moderns, Jean-Jacques Rousseau (1762 cited in Scott 2012). One of Rousseau's contemporaries wrote that individuals 'exist independently of society; they form its necessary elements, and they enter it in order to put themselves . . . under the protection of . . . [the] laws to which they sacrifice their liberty' (Turgot, cited in Lukes 1973: 77). Individuals have their own independent consciousness that arises naturally from birth and that allows them to determine their own wants and needs, and to be the best judges of their own interests.

This way of understanding individuals attracted some vigorous criticism from others who also subscribed to Enlightenment ideas and ideals. The most significant of these were Europeans writing mainly in the 19th century, and at the heart of their critique was the concept of society, or the social. The idea of society had been recognised by the early moderns but mainly as an agglomeration of individuals who came together – forming an association – by way of a *contract* or agreement from which they would all benefit by doing so (see, for example, Locke in Shapiro 2003, Smith 1776 in Sutherland 2008, Rousseau 1762 in Scott 2012). Underpinning this idea was the belief that individuals were part of nature and that nature was a tough place to be if you were on your own or living in small family groups. Society was invented by individuals wanting to come in out of the cold of nature, as it were. Among the most trenchant critics of this idea was one of the earlier sociologists, the French scholar Emile Durkheim (1858–1917), and a legally trained German social theorist living in mid-19th century London, Karl Marx (1818–83). They proposed that understanding individuals as being naturally all the same – outside and prior to social life – stripped them of their concreteness, turning them into abstractions that failed to represent individuals as 'real' people engaged in living and doing things in varied and specific kinds of circumstances. Marx proposed that thinking about human beings in this way made them *abstract individuals* (Marx 1845) who did not, in fact, exist in reality.

Durkheim and Marx developed a radically different take on individuals that was forged in the turbulence of industrialising (see below) Europe in the 19th century. Individuals did not spring from nature and enter society as fully formed human beings, they insisted. The social was always ever-present, and human animals were born into and transformed by it into human beings. The kinds of human beings they became depended on the kinds of societies that produced and raised them. For both Marx and Durkheim (1895: 103), society or the social was not 'a mere sum of individuals'. It was evident, they wrote, in the specific *patterns* of collective life they identified in 19th-century industrialising Europe. Clearly, there was more happening than could be explained by individual psychology or the simple aggregation of individual motivations and actions. But what was it?

Industrialisation, social practices and the division of labour

The seismic reverberations of 19th-century industrialisation involved rapid and irrevocable changes in the day-to-day circumstances and lives of working people that occurred on an unprecedented scale. This transformation began in Britain as early as the 16th century and spread to other European countries from the 17th century onwards (Hill 1969). Among the most dramatically affected were the landless rural villagers of 18th-century Britain who were no longer able to support themselves and their families as the farming land they had inhabited for centuries was converted for other purposes: primarily agricultural and pastoral production for sale on a *market*, but also game parks and other recreational activity (Hobsbawm 1969a, Thompson 1993). They crowded haphazardly into the towns and cities of England and Scotland to work in the mills and factories around which they took up residence. Much has been written of the hellish existence that the many hundreds of thousands involved in this development eked out. Manchester – England's second-largest city after London in the 19th century – was second to none in producing the opportunities for such a life, as the following sickeningly illustrates.

Manchester, England, 1844

In 1844, a young German businessman, Frederick Engels, visited Manchester to observe the social conditions of what was considered then to be the world's most advanced industrialised centre. Engels subsequently wrote a detailed description of what he had witnessed and expressed his disbelief and disgust at what he had seen. One of the most graphic excerpts from his account centred on the city's River Irk. According to Engels, the banks of the Irk were very high – up to 30 feet on the southern side. Yet, three rows of houses could be seen planted along the banks, with the lowest rising 'directly out of the river' (Engels 1844/1950: 48). Interspersed among the houses were mills. The overall picture was one of crowded and knotted chaos. Meanwhile, Engels reported, emanating from the main street was a labyrinth of covered passages that spilled into courts, many leading down to the river. The filth and grime of the passageways were even worse in the dwellings located in the courts. 'In one of these ... there [stood] directly at the entrance ... a privy without a door, so dirty that the inhabitants [could] pass into and out of the court only by passing through foul pools of stagnant urine and excrement' (Engels 1844/1950: 48). On the river, there was a number of tanneries polluting the neighbourhood with the foul stench of animal decay. Below the Ducie Bridge, which spanned the Irk, narrow, dirty stairs, heaped with refuse and filth, were the only means of entry to the houses. The view from the bridge was typical of the whole district. At the bottom seeped 'the narrow, coal-black, foul-smelling Irk', full of debris and garbage, which it [deposited] on its banks. Nearby drains and all the waste from tanneries, bone mills and gas works found their way into the Irk – choked further by 'the contents of all the neighbouring sewers and privies...' (Engels 1844/1950: 49-50).

The dwellings along the river comprised small, single-storied, one-roomed huts with dirt floors. Kitchen, living and sleeping-room were all in one. In such places, which generally were no more than five feet long by six feet wide, one might find two beds, 'which, with a staircase and chimney-place, filled the room'. Garbage and offal lay everywhere outside front doors and over walkways. So thick was this carpet of filth that 'any sort of pavement' could not be seen but only felt in different places as one walked.

The mess of one-roomed, rickety holes along the banks of the Irk was virtually uninhabitable – with the degree of filth and squalor largely inescapable, both inside and outside such dwellings. Sanitation facilities were so rare that they either filled up every day or were too scarce for most of the inhabitants to use. The landlords, however, saw no shame in letting such premises despite the fact that the floors of many of them stood 'at least two feet below the low-water level of the Irk that [flowed] not six feet away from them...' (Engels 1844/1950: 51–2)

The horrific environmental and living conditions depicted by Engels in his eye-witness account – and subsequently confirmed by historians (Hobsbawm 1969b: 15–17) – provide graphic evidence of the dehumanising and destructive character of early industrialisation. Similar conditions were reported in other industrialising towns and cities in England and Scotland, indicating an identifiable pattern of human existence. The replication of such conditions was accompanied by people's ways of living – or *social practices* – that grew remarkably more similar across the industrialising landscape. Regional variations persisted but there emerged an increasing homogeneity in the activities of everyday life that revealed new and collective patterns of practices. For example, the woollen, linen and leather clothing that rural villagers typically wore, providing some protection against the cold and wet (Hill 1969), disappeared as they swarmed into the manufacturing towns and cities. Men, women and children were everywhere clothed in cotton – dresses, shirts, trousers, jackets, coats – that all too quickly turned to rags (Engels 1844/1950: 66–7). Many were barefoot, especially women and children. Diet consisted mainly of bread, cheese, porridge and potatoes, with better-paid workers and families, who all were earning something, able to eat meat daily. Starvation was widespread (Engels 1844/1950:73–4). The affordability of working people's food generally relied on acceptance of the very poorest-quality produce – much of which was contaminated, rancid, stale, old, decaying and withered. The *Liverpool Mercury* (cited in Engels 1844/1950: 70) reported in 1844 that adulteration of foodstuffs was endemic: 'The refuse of soap-boiling establishments...is mixed with other things and sold as sugar...Cocoa is often adulterated with fine brown earth, treated with fat to render it more easily mistakable for real cocoa...[P]ort-wine is manufactured outright [out of alcohol, dye-stuffs etc.].'

These patterns of social practice were directly linked to the very low incomes that working people received – a key feature of the expansion of a social practice that had prevailed in Britain at least since the 14th century (MacFarlane 1978: 152) – *work for wages* or *employment*. Prior to industrialisation most people did not depend on employment – or selling their labour on a *market* – to survive. They *subsisted*, living and working in households and villages, and producing things for their own use; all largely according to the rhythms of the sun and the seasons (Thompson 1980). Industrialisation established workplaces that separated people from their households, intensifying their hours of work and imposing strict disciplines and harsh penalties for failure to comply with them (Thompson 1980).

Though the spread of a labour *market* and work for wages did not occur at the same pace and with the same intensity across the country (Pahl 1984), it became the main type of work for men, women and children forced off land turned to industrialised production. By the mid-19th century, Britons were employed in a wide range of occupations and industries, not only manufacturing. Some women, for example, remained engaged in agriculture in rural areas – the main occupation of working women in the 18th century – but throughout the 19th century one-third of urban working women sought employment as domestic servants (Pahl 1984). Many working people, uprooted from permanent residence anywhere, made their wages in hawking goods and services of an extraordinary variety wherever they could in urban street stalls and markets, as Henry Mayhew's book, *London's Labour and the London Poor* (1861), vividly recounts.

Nineteenth-century industrialisation in Britain, then, produced new and diverse social practices that were patterned in a number of ways. Yet, it was the pattern of practices related to employment and the *division of labour* that sociologists such as Durkheim (1893) and Marx identified as the cornerstone of industrialised social life and the foundation upon which the distinction between pre-industrial and industrialised life was built. Neither Durkheim nor Marx, however, invented the term 'division of labour'. Like 'the individual', it was a product of modernist European thinking, arising primarily as a way of describing the ways in which people were increasingly *specialising* in producing things and trading or exchanging them with one another. One of the most-renowned popularisers of the idea was an English economist called Adam Smith (1763/1978), who believed that division of labour was the motor of human prosperity and progress because of the great increase in the quantity of work and goods that resulted. In a famous passage, Smith described the processes involved in the industrialised division of labour in relation to making pins:

> One man draws out the wire, another straightens it, a third cuts it, a fourth points it, a fifth grinds it at the top for . . . the head; to make the head requires two or three distinct operations . . . [M]aking a pin [in fact] . . . is divided into eighteen distinct operations . . . [each usually] performed by distinct hands. (Smith 1763/1978)

The social: Structure, dynamics and power

For Durkheim (1893), there was no doubt that the rampant growth of the industrialised division of labour had caused enormous upheaval and imposed insufferable social costs of the kind illustrated above. However, the occupational specialisation that revolutionised work regimens brought with it a major human advance. It established the conditions for greater individual difference at the same time as increasing people's dependence on each other, because survival demanded exchange of goods and services. According to Durkheim, this was a win–win situation: people's individuality and independence could flourish at the same time as interdependence – or the *social order* and stability – could be strengthened. The industrialised division of labour produced what Durkheim called a new *solidarity* among people that enabled everyday life to keep ticking over or functioning in the interests of everybody – although some would benefit more from it than others because of natural differences that would translate into occupational differences and rewards intrinsic to the new order.

It is evident that, from Durkheim's perspective, the social was a reality brought into being by the actions and interactions of individuals that could not be 'accounted for in terms of the properties of individual actors' (Coser 1971: 130). It was a 'system formed by (individuals') association [and] represent[ing] a specific reality which has its own characteristics' (Durkheim 1895: 103). Though produced by multiple actors engaged in diverse and complex actions, the social was more than the sum of such actors and their actions. This 'system' exercised power over individuals that obliged them to act in ways that were not of their own making. According to Durkheim, it had a dynamic of its own that was like all earthly organisms – both plant and animal. Conceived of in this way, society was driven towards survival through the combined functioning of all of its parts.

The London-based Marx, writing and publishing almost a half century before Durkheim, had a very different take on Adam Smith's industrialised division of labour and, more significantly, on the social and how it worked. Marx was a close friend of the German businessman who penned the account of the grimy grisliness of industrialising Manchester previously described. Their first-hand knowledge of the industrialised division of labour and the social conditions that accompanied it left little room for any favourable view of its contribution to the advancement of the values and ideals of the Enlightenment, especially those associated with individual freedom and equality. In fact, they believed that the industrialisation they witnessed made the achievement of Enlightenment ideals impossible. Yet, it was not industrialisation itself that was the main problem. There were other social dynamics operating. Marx's account of what these were and how they worked produced a new and original approach to the social, as the following outlines.

Marx, like Durkheim, understood society as a process that obliged individuals to do things that were not entirely of their own making (Marx 1852/1963). However, for Marx, this dynamic was not generated by some kind of spontaneous organic force that sought its own survival and reproduction in the interests of everybody. Rather, it arose through patterns of social practice established over time – *social structures* – into which people were born and with which they were obliged to interact in their everyday lives. So society was something that human beings themselves produced (or did) but not in any random way, nor according to the conscious, collective wills of individuals, as influential 18th-century European thinkers proposed. The social was inescapably a legacy of past human action combined with contemporary collective practice. Most significantly, society and its defining patterns of practice were primarily what happened in response to what Marx proposed was the overriding necessity of all human existence: the need to eat and the practices involved in enabling human beings to do so. How human beings organised this *material production* was the foundation of all other social structures and the practices that brought them into being. Marx called it the *base* structure and its mode of operation basically shaped the possibilities for what collectivities of people could do in the rest of their lives. Marx developed his account of society based on reading and analysis of a wide collection of sources – historical, anthropological, economic, scientific, journalistic and so on – and published in diverse, mainly European, languages. So, unlike the emergent practices of the physical sciences, where direct empirical observation of matter and energy was central, Marx's practice for identifying and understanding how the social worked mainly involved the collection and analysis of documentary sources about human social practice.

According to Marx, the industrialised division of labour described by Adam Smith was undoubtedly a tour de force in human development, particularly in terms of the sheer size and scale of material goods that could enrich human lives. The problem was, however, that this way of organising people to produce things – in highly specialised occupations and industries – dehumanised those who did the work involved in the process. Not only were workers subjected to boring repetition, denying autonomy and opportunities for self-development as imagined by Enlightenment thinking, their very dignity as human beings with *rights* to basic survival was compromised by dangerous working conditions and processes. Further, the wages that most workers received in return barely enabled them to survive, as shown in the Manchester case study.

At the same time, the minority of people who owned and ran the processes of industrialised production – the mills, the factories, the mines, the farms and so on – were not only shielded from their harms but also received most of the material benefits, primarily the *profits* they made when the products were sold at market. These profits could only be made, Marx proposed, by *exploitation* of those who did the work for the owners and managers: in other words, by paying the workers who produced the goods only a fraction of the money for which they were sold at market – or *wages*. In so doing, the owners and managers were *extracting a surplus* from the labour of those whom they employed, keeping it for themselves. Needless to say, such a *mode of production*, as Marx called it, and the practices through which it operated – particularly in relation to minority ownership of the materials needed to produce things – meant that the *idea* of the equal worth of individuals and their innate dignity remained precisely that. Far from advancing solidarity among people, as Durkheim suggested, the industrialised division of labour served as a mechanism for systematically creating a social structure characterised by *hierarchy* or *social division*: between those forced to be employed, earning wages for a living, and those who were not. What drove it, as Marx argued, was the relentless pursuit of profit and its accumulation as capital. To the extent that it persisted, workers and owners were inextricably caught up in a relationship of interdependence, but one that necessarily yielded unequal returns to the two participants. Advances in the material benefits of one (wages or profits) could only be obtained at the expense of the other's, so *conflict* was intrinsic to the relationship. Marx called this pattern of practice or social structure *class*. Two distinct social groups were brought into being as a consequence: the proletariat (or working class) and the bourgeoisie (or those owning the productive means and capital). So class referred both to the structure (or relationship) *and* the groups – or classes – involved. Intrinsic to it was *power*, understood here to mean the capacity of one group to dominate and subordinate another, forcing it to do things that brought greater benefits to the dominant than the subordinate (Lukes 2005).

The 19th-century novelist Emile Zola (1885) wrote contemptuously of this polarised relationship and dynamic with respect to the coal fields of France, as the following extract shows.

> ... [T]he Gregoires had maintained an obstinate faith in their mine ... [W]ith [their] religious faith was mixed profound gratitude towards an investment which for a century had supported the family in doing nothing. It was like a divinity of their own ... the benefactor of the hearth, lulling them in their great bed of idleness, fattening them at their gluttonous table. From father to son it had gone on ... [Their wealth] seemed to them ... sheltered in the earth, from which a race of miners, generations of starving people, extracted it for them, a little every day, as they needed it. (Zola 1994: 79–80)

Fast-forwarding to the early 21st century

More than 150 years later, most of the world's industrialised production for profit – particularly in manufacturing and mining – has moved to China, South Asia, South-east Asia and sub-Saharan Africa. At the same time, the countries in which the wealthy minority of the global population resides are often referred to as 'post-industrial societies'. Can these 19th-century ideas about society and how it works, then, help us to make sense of and understand the social in contemporary settings and on a global scale? The short answer is yes and no. What both Durkheim and Marx proposed that remains absolutely as relevant now as then is the idea that the social is more than the sum of individuals, obliging both individuals and groups to act in ways that are not reducible to psychological motivations. The social, then, exceeds individuals but, as Durkheim and Marx also emphasised, it precedes individuals in the sense that we are born into it. A further compelling contribution relevant to understanding the contemporary social is Marx's idea of human action and behaviour as practice, and the social as a collective accomplishment of it.

Some sociologists continue to embrace an approach informed by Durkheim's thinking – *functionalism* – that society exists through a drive towards integration of its diverse and even conflicted components into an ongoing and functioning whole (Colomy 1991). Others subscribe to Marx's idea that *class conflict* and *struggle* continue to lie at the heart of the social, consistently creating inequality, crisis and instability, and on a global scale – albeit in ways that need to be understood in contemporary historical contexts (see Burawoy 2000). Many, however, have rejected the 19th-century European formulations of 'dead White men' such as Durkheim and Marx, in turn devising wholly new or radically modified approaches. At the heart of much of the new thinking about the social is that it is far more complex than 19th-century approaches suggested and that the vast global changes in the social that have occurred since then demand conceptual innovations and previously marginalised voices to understand them. For example, there is more to the foundation and operation of contemporary social structure than the economic division of labour and its relationship to the pursuit of profit and accumulation of capital. There are also multiple ways in which power can be understood as operating in and animating social practice. Over a century of social research into an astonishing array of practices in innumerable locations, and critical reflection about them, have refreshed sociological concepts and enabled them to continue to have explanatory force. One of the most significant advances in this regard is the challenge to the *determinism* of 19th-century ideas about social structure and of the relationship of *human agency* (see below) to it.

This book reflects these developments particularly with respect to how we might understand social structure and power. As the following chapters show, social structures are multiple but some are more significant than others. Further, while they exert enormous influence over what we do in our day-to-day lives, they do so in ways that are far less mechanical and predictable than what our 19th-century forebears proposed. As Australian sociologist Raewyn Connell (2002) has written, social structures are definitely patterned (not random), extensive (not sporadic or episodic) and enduring (not ephemeral) social relations but they cannot exist separately from practices. Structures such as class 'do not continue, cannot be "enduring", unless they are reconstituted from moment to moment in social action' (Connell 2002: 55). As such, they do not cause or determine practices, or 'how people or groups act' (Connell 2002: 55). They define possibilities for and constraints on practice. This approach to social structure renders it more *dynamic*. Though involving fixity and durability, social structure is simultaneously a process comprised of human activity. From this perspective, what many sociologists have characterised as something independent of structure – collective human agency – is indivisibly embedded in or intrinsic to structures of social practice. In other words, social structures do not operate without human agency. How they do so is one of the great pursuits of sociology.

The focus of this book is in identifying what the main processes are in producing social inequality and global health inequities, and how they work in doing so. Its main lens derives from a long tradition in the social sciences, called 'critical sociology' or 'critical theory'. Central to this tradition is the use of a combination of social science disciplines – history, political economy, geography, social policy, political theory and so on. As significant is a specific sense of purpose associated with the whole enterprise. It is not simply to describe, analyse and understand the social but, rather, the *inequalities and injustices* that arise from it, and how they may be addressed and redressed through social action. As this book explains, the indivisibility of health and the social – or the marriage between the two – means that the global project to 'close the gap' in health demands a thoroughgoing understanding of the social divisions that cause it.

Conclusions

This chapter introduces and explains the idea of society or the social from a sociological perspective. It does so by telling a particular story that is set largely in a time and places that no longer exist but that continue to resonate in all of our lives. At the heart of the story is a European development called the Enlightenment, advancing a new idea that humans are individuals with innate dignity and worth, and able to be the best judges of how to be in the world. One of the most radical features of this new thinking is that *all* humans are individuals and, as such, equal but unique. Paradoxically, this idea gradually spread across the globe as Europeans colonised much of the world, ruthlessly supplanting Indigenous ideas and ways of living with their own. According to Enlightenment thinkers, society happened as a result of individuals rationally agreeing to sacrifice some of their individual freedom to come together for their individual betterment in the face of a hostile nature.

Not all of them agreed, however. Others who lived and studied in the 18th and 19th centuries bearing witness to the upheavals of the industrial revolution in Europe had different ideas about the social. One of these, French sociologist Emile Durkheim, argued that these interactions were subject to a 'system' established by previous human interaction that obliged individuals to act in ways that were not of their own making. This system was the social and, basically, with the new division of labour established by industrialisation, it operated towards its perpetuation so that all might benefit, albeit in different and unequal ways because of natural disparities among individuals. Karl Marx, a further analyst of the social, had a very different view of how the social worked. He understood the social as a creation of collective human practice that became embedded over time in the practice of subsequent generations of people. The social was something that preceded individual action but required its enactment in the present in order to exist. The ways in which this process was patterned determined subsequent human action. Far from advancing individuality and solidarity as Durkheim suggested, for Marx the industrialised division of labour under capitalism in the 18th and 19th centuries produced thoroughgoing social division and conflict based on economic exploitation of the majority by a property owning minority. It was this division and its associated struggles – called 'class' – that comprised the heart of the social, determining the fates and fortunes of the individuals involved in the process. Enlightenment aspirations for individual freedom and equality – and societal harmony – were rendered chimerical as a result.

One of the most useful tools of this 19th-century sociological legacy is that of social structure and power. As the remaining chapters of this book show, there is no single, central social structure, such as class, as Marx suggested. Rather, there are several, and they shape our lives and our fortunes, including our health, in extraordinarily powerful ways. Recent advances in sociological thinking now enable us to understand social structure in ways that bring day-to-day social action and the sediments of past collective practice together. Social structure is an enduring pattern of practice – a process – in which groups and individuals engage, always drawing on past patterns of practice, but forging possibilities and constraints for future action. It is the *combination* of these dynamic social processes, with their resonances of the past intrinsic to their enactment, that comprise society. It is their distinctive combination and differentiation from others that allow us to distinguish how particular societies work and how they affect our embodiment, especially that associated with health.

Questions for discussion

1   What does the slave trade that operated in the Atlantic between Africa and the British colonies of North America in the 18th century tell us about prevailing understandings of the individual at the time?
2   What was the Enlightenment and how did it affect thinking about human being and action at around the same time as the Atlantic slave trade in the 18th century?
3   What distinguishes pre-modernity from modernity?
4   How did the early moderns of the 18th century conceive of society? Why were 19th-century contributors to understanding the social critical of their 18th-century predecessors' formulations?

5   What were some of the patterns of social conditions and practices in the industrialising towns of 19th-century Britain that were dehumanising and dangerous?

6   What was the industrialised 'division of labour' and why did Durkheim and Marx think it was significant?

7   Marx had a specific approach to understanding what the social is and how it works. What do you understand as its key features? How did Marx conceptualise social structure and how it operated? Why has it been criticised as deterministic?

8   In what sense can Durkheim's approach to the social be described as functionalist?

9   Social structure:
    a   What do you understand by the term 'social structure'?
    b   What does it mean to say that social structures are dynamic?
    c   What are the advantages of understanding social structures in this way?
    d   Can you think of an example to illustrate dynamic social structure?

3 Class and health

Overview

- What is the social gradient in health? What are some of the key indicators of socio-economic status (SES) used to identify it?

- What is the relationship between SES and social resources? What kinds of health disparities can it explain?

- What is specific to class as a domain of social practice? What does it seek to explain in relation to health?

- What is the division of labour and what role does it play in producing class?

- How does the ownership and control of the resources needed for producing and distributing goods and services generate class?

- What are representational practices and discourses? What role do they play in class dynamics?

- How does class get into peoples' bodies as health and illness?

California, United States, 2013

As one of this year's memorable episodes of the television program 'Keeping Up With the Kardashians' showed, Kim Kardashian's pregnancy and baby appeared to be in crisis. Less than a week later, Kardashian and partner Kanye West had their first child, delivering a very happy ending to the medical drama.

On a flight during which Kardashian experienced unexpected distress, the reality star reported that she had 'never experienced pain like this in her life', and was rushed to her doctor. 'The episode offered a behind-the-scenes look at her personal anxieties and fears for what has been a very public pregnancy'.

Kardashian's mother, Kris Jenner, raced to the doctor's office, where she found her daughter in agony and sobbing on the examination table. I will 'never do this again' Kardashian vowed. Believing the problem to have been appendicitis, the family was worried that Kardashian would have to undergo surgical intervention. Fortunately, the pain was the result of a stomach infection. Her fever raised serious concerns for the baby's condition but the doctor found a healthy heartbeat, indicating that there were no problems.

'Baby Kimye was born on Saturday, about five weeks early, and the Kardashians have been uncharacteristically quiet about the details of the birth and the baby' (*Huffington Post* 2013).

As the reality television show 'Keeping Up With the Kardashians' has revealed to the world since its inception in 2007, the Kardashians are rich and glamorous North Americans. They are portrayed in the television series as 'being themselves' at home, in their business lives, on holidays, going shopping and so on – and in the opulent settings they typically inhabit. Apart from the birthing crisis described above, the Kardashians have not had any other medical encounters on television. They and their friends, in fact, enjoy very good health and, when they face a 'serious health scare', as 30-year-old Kim Kardashian allegedly did with her pregnancy, they have immediate access to high-tech specialist medical care (see Chapter 8). Obstetric care in the United States, like its counterparts in other wealthy OECD countries like Australia, is especially renowned for its rates of technical interventions such as caesarean sections, reaching an all-time high of 32 per cent of all births in 2007 (Menacker and Hamilton 2010), and remaining at around this level since. In the United States, caesarean sections are performed for a number of reasons, but 'maternal choice' is on the increase, generating widespread 'chosen prematurity' (Menacker and Hamilton 2010).

At the global level, premature birth is not usually associated with choice. It is more commonly related to perinatal and infant mortality, and lifelong impairment. According to the social determinants of health approach, it is also one of the strongest indicators of poverty and low socio-economic status (SES), and occurs much more commonly in the world's low to middle-income countries than its rich ones (WHO 2013d). It still affects women and their babies in high-income countries, as Kim Kardashian's experience shows, but not usually among the wealthy and privileged, like the members of the Kardashian family in California. Around 12 per cent of all births in the United States are premature (Norwitz 2014), of which most (80 per cent) are spontaneous, but they are significantly more likely to happen to pregnant women from the 'lowest SES bands', especially if they are African-American (see Chapter 5) – not their high SES counterparts (US Centers for Disease Control and Prevention 2013).

Why might this be the case? How do SES differences – as also briefly discussed in Chapter 1 – get 'under the skin' or into people's bodies, producing health inequity? This chapter focuses on addressing these questions by engaging with the sociological concept of *class* introduced in the previous chapter. It does so with close attention to the bodily realities of class in everyday life, specifically the ways in which the social processes involved materialise in our bodies as 'health'. First, however, we turn to the social dimensions of class. As we saw in the previous chapter, class was central to Karl Marx's story about the social, especially social hierarchy, conflict and inequality. But Marx is not the only one for whom this concept has proved useful – indeed, central – in understanding social division. There are innumerable sociologists who review and discuss class (see, for example, Wright 2005, Giddens and Sutton 2014, Van Krieken et al. 2014). This chapter submits an account of class that focuses on the relationship between SES indicators and health inequities – both within countries and on a global scale. Such explanations – or conceptual tools – are critical in shaping both our understandings of social problems, such as health inequities, and our actions to address and redress them. First, however, we revisit SES and its relationship to health differences and disparities.

SES and health disparities

Most of what we know about SES and health disparities is drawn from databases and research conducted in high-income countries, especially the United States and the United Kingdom. There are some significant exceptions, and these are very valuable, as the findings from a study on income inequalities and mortality rates within countries globally, presented below, show. However, our knowledge and understanding of health disparities and SES within low and middle-income countries are much more limited. As we saw in Chapter 1, the main indicators of SES used in conjunction with health are income, education and occupational status. The most commonly used health indicators in relation to mapping the health effects of SES inequalities are life expectancy and mortality rates, but rates of disease, injury and disability are often also included. SES indicators are closely intertwined – or interdependent – in their health effects (Lahelma et al. 2004). Thus, a measure of the relationship between one of them, such as income differentials in a large population, and a major health indicator, such as their life expectancy rates, often serves as a good tool for approximating the overall magnitude of their health disparities by SES. Nevertheless, combining SES indicators and matching them with a health indicator such as life expectancy is a more 'robust' basis upon which to measure the pattern of health disparities and social inequality. Figure 3.1 illustrates the application of this latter approach to documenting inequalities in life expectancy by SES of the total population in the United States over a 20-year period from 1980 to 2000. The authors of the study combined key indicators of SES selected from education, occupation, wealth, income distribution, unemployment

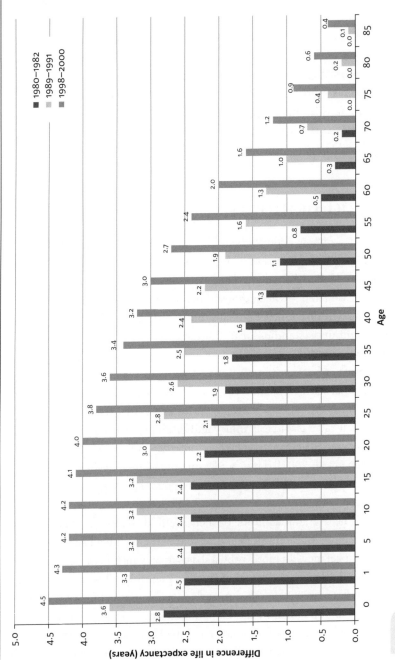

FIGURE 3.1 Inequalities in life expectancy between the least-deprived and most-deprived socio-economic groups, United States, 1980–2000
Source: Singh & Siahpush 2006: 975.

TABLE 3.1 *Standardised mortality ratios in the United States by educational level for men and women aged 35–75 years, 1983–2003*

	LESS THAN HIGH SCHOOL	HIGH SCHOOL	SOME COLLEGE	COLLEGE
Women	1.37	0.93	0.81	0.65
Men	1.32	1.02	0.91	0.62

Source: Compiled from Cristia 2009: 32–3.

rate, poverty rate and housing quality to create an index of 'socio-economic deprivation' in order to measure socio-economic inequality and its relationship to life expectancy (Singh and Siapush 2006). Figure 3.1 shows the differences in life expectancy by age between the 'the least deprived' – those with the highest SES – and 'the most deprived' – those with the lowest SES. These differences are presented over three time periods (indicated by the different columns in the graph), showing an increase in the inequalities in life expectancy by the number of years for all age groups from 1980 to 2000. For example, the difference in life expectancy between 20-year-olds in the United States who fell into the lowest SES band (or 'most deprived') and the highest SES band (or 'least deprived') between 1980 and 2000 increased from 2.2 to 4 years. This trend applied to every age group, but there was a gradient indicating that health disparities by SES were greatest among Americans under one year of age and reducing with increased age – a trend that characterises most OECD countries (Dorling, Mitchell and Pearce 2007). It is evident then that health disparities in the United States, as measured by the relationship between life expectancy and a combination of key SES indicators, are an established feature of the health landscape in that country.

Standardised mortality ratios (SMRs) are considered among the most accurate mortality measures and are widely used as an indicator of health disparity by SES. Table 3.1 shows how greater levels or years of education among both men and women (aged 35–75 years) in the United States correspond with a decline in the SMR. The SMRs in Table 3.1 express the numbers of women and men between the ages of 35 and 75 years, over a 20-year period and with varying degrees of education, who died as a percentage of the total American populations of men and women respectively in this age range who died at that time. The SMR for women with less than high school was 1.37. This is significantly over 100, meaning that, on the whole, many more women with less than a high school education and between the ages of 35 and 75 years (37 per cent more) died in the United States than the overall national death rate of this age group of women over this time. At the same time, the SMR of 0.65 for women with college education in this age range indicates that 35 per cent fewer of them died than might have been expected from the national figures. The SMRs for men indicate a similar trend but the differences in SMRs between men and women are greater for those with 'high school' and 'some college' education than they are for men and women with 'less than high school' and 'college' education. These variations raise questions about how *gender* interacts with SES to produce health disparities – an issue explored further in Chapter 4.

Income inequalities provide a further major indicator of health disparities within countries across the globe. Based on 2002 data, a British study of mortality rates and income differentials by age and gender in 126 countries, selected from the full spectrum of low, middle and high-income countries, found that income level had a major effect on mortality in every country (Dorling, Mitchell and Pearse 2007). Lower incomes were associated with significantly higher death rates everywhere, and were most pronounced for people aged 15–29 years and 25–39 years. 'This relation was especially strong among the poorest countries in Africa' (Dorling et al. 2007: 1) but widespread throughout the world at marginally lower intensity. As the study's authors noted, 'some 3.5 billion people, more than half the world population, survive on the equivalent, or less, of what $10 in the US would buy a day' (Dorling et al. 2007: 3). The study concluded that:

> ...social inequalities as reflected through unequal incomes are damaging to health for those living in both rich and poor nations, and the direct mechanisms for such damage are likely to vary by area...However, the underlying mechanism may be similar – that, because humans are social animals, human health is best protected when people cooperate (rather than compete with each other). (Dorling et al. 2007: 4)

Such a conclusion has significant implications for this chapter because, as explained further on, class is a major dynamic of social division involving relations of competition and conflict between groups of people. Cooperation features in the process but is more common *within* groups than between them. Before moving to this discussion, however, we turn to a further SES indicator – occupational status, or 'employment grade' – and its relationship to health differences and disparities. Here, the results of a famous British research project – the Whitehall investigations – remain the 'gold standard' for demonstrating the powerful correlation between differences in position in an occupational hierarchy and mortality disparities.

The Whitehall studies

The first Whitehall study was established in 1967 and included 18 000 men in the British Civil Service. Its results showed that men in the lowest employment grades had greater rates of premature mortality than their counterparts in the highest grades. Yet, the differences were not attributable to well-known risk factors, such as smoking.

In 1985, Professor Sir Michael Marmot and his University College London (UCL) team set up the Whitehall II study to determine the factors that might contribute to the social gradient in death and disease identified in the previous study, and to include women. The study proceeded between 1985 and 1988 with a baseline survey of 10 308 non-industrial civil servants from the London-based offices of 20 civil service departments. They ranged in age from 35 to 55 years. Women comprised around one-third of the survey participants. This first phase of the study required that participants undertake a medical examination and complete a questionnaire. A further 10 phases of data collection have followed since then (UCL Research Department of Epidemiology and Public Health 2013).

A follow-up study by the Whitehall II team showed an 'inverse association' between occupational status and average mortality at age 40–64 years among men working in the British Civil Service between 1967 and 1970 (Marmot and Shipley 1996). Occupational status was based on a hierarchy of four categories. From the highest to lowest these were administrative, professional/executive, clerical and 'other'. Those in the administrative category had about half the average mortality at age 40–64 yrs, while the office support staff who made up the 'other' had about twice the average. Thus, there was a four-fold difference between those at the bottom and those at the top (Ferrie 2004).

As the data from these various studies show, the best life expectancy and mortality outcomes are strongly associated with a combination of high-income levels, high educational levels and employment in 'high-status' occupations. At the same time, the worst health outcome measures correspond with a combination of low income and education levels, and employment in low-status occupations. These correlations, as epidemiologists propose, indicate a *social health gradient* that prevails virtually universally within countries and between them, as we saw in Chapter 1. The social gradient of health refers to inequalities in health outcomes based on SES. Globally, lower SES is associated with poorer health (Marmot and Wilkinson 2006). The following section explains how SES is inextricably related to social resources that are critical for health.

SES and unequal access to social resources

In sociological terms, SES indicators represent measurable inequalities in people's *access to the social resources they need for health*. Hierarchical access to these resources produces unequal health fortunes, as illustrated by the differential health outcome measures presented above. The following summarises and explains the main social resources associated with health.

Material resources are critical to health. They encompass anything of material value that people can use for their benefit. Wealth and income usually qualify as the most significant. There are various definitions of wealth according to economists, but it commonly includes two kinds of assets. 'Non-financial assets' are those that do not produce income, such as homes, real estate, vehicles and jewellery. 'Financial assets', by comparison, generate income and include savings, bonds, shares and retirement pensions.

Symbolic resources are also vital to people's health because they too involve the delivery of human benefits. They are generally less concrete and often more complex than material resources. Educational qualifications and occupational status are indicators of symbolic resources that exert major health effects (as we have seen above) and, like wealth and income, are measurable on a population basis. Yet, educational qualifications and occupational status are not the same as the resources they represent. While occupational status, for example, indicates a position in a hierarchy, as we saw in the Whitehall studies, it reveals nothing of the actual symbolic benefits delivered to those who 'occupy' such a position. The symbolic resource that comes with occupational status is basically *recognition* (Honneth 1995, 2007) – or *not* – of people's worth or value that derives from the position they occupy. Occupational value is recognised through the conferral and distribution of autonomy and control over work and others within an occupational hierarchy. Occupation of a superior position, or high occupational status, represents greater recognition through autonomy and control, while relegation to an inferior occupational location – low occupational status – reflects limited or no recognition and tight control and supervision.

Educational participation also operates as a major symbolic resource insofar as it is usually required for recognition as worthy of entering 'superior' occupational positions. However, the benefits it delivers are not confined to occupational recognition. Participating in education is one of the chief mechanisms by which we are enabled to take part in the *symbolic processes* of social life. Education generates capacities, knowledges and intellectual technologies – or 'know-how' resources – for participating in and understanding the diverse *symbolic* dimensions of everyday life, such as what things mean, how they work, why, with what effects and in whose interests. They are critical to navigating everyday life, both individually and collectively – and they affect health in ways that remain poorly understood. For example, increments in levels of education among women everywhere in the world correspondingly reduce rates of child mortality, independent of women's occupation and income (Fischetti 2011).

Sociologists suggest some symbolic resources have greater social legitimacy than others; for example, the knowledges and languages of the professions compared with those of, say, criminal gangs; or the knowledge and language of 'haute cuisine' compared to that of frozen dinners and fast food. The symbolic resources with higher social value can be accumulated as 'symbolic capital' (Bourdieu and Wacquant 1992), hence making explicit the *power* such resources embody. The symbolic resources associated with education are closely aligned to a further source of widespread human benefit.

Agentic resources enable people collectively and individually to *act on* and *influence* their everyday lives, and are inextricably linked to *participation* that confers rewards and satisfactions critical to people's health (Labonte and Laverack 2001, Laverack 2006, Rifkin 2003). Prominent examples of such resources include participation in employment and workplace organisation, in associations with others (such as religious organisations, trade unions, sport and leisure groups, community based organisations and social movements), in political life (such as voting, membership of political parties and lobby groups) and in institutions of the state (such as parliaments). Among public health scholars, agentic resources are commonly referred to as 'empowerment' (Labonte and Laverack 2001).

From a social resource-based perspective, then, health is made scarce or abundant according to the magnitude of access to material, symbolic and agentic resources: in general, the greater the access, the better the health, and vice versa. As such, the correlations that proliferate in the epidemiological literature are a kind of quantitative 'short hand' for representing this relationship. As explained further throughout this book, access to material, symbolic and agentic resources is linked to health, and not only in securing day-to-day embodied survival. Such access is linked to the benefits that people can accumulate over time in their bodies as health – in other words, as healthy adults and older people (Blane 2006). The following explains how class is one of the key social processes responsible for the unequal access to social resources indicated by SES differences and the health disparities that accompany them.

Class: A specific domain of social relations and practices

Chapter 2 emphasised that class is a social process – a structure of practices involved in producing social division and inequality. It is not the only such process involved, as subsequent chapters show. There is a number of *domains of social practice* responsible for producing social inequalities and health inequities, such as gender, ethnicity, indigeneity and the state, but each is distinctive. *What distinguishes class from the others is that it centres on a process with several key features: the production and distribution of goods and services, ownership/control of resources required for the purpose and their symbolisation.* It is how this process is socially organised that determines whether it creates a division among people called 'class'. If the process is organised in such a way that class does result, then some will enjoy much greater access to material, symbolic and agentic resources at the expense of the vast majority. Class, then, always involves *power*. This chapter proposes that the following structures of practice and how they are combined are foundational in producing class and establishing it as a social domain distinct from other generators of social hierarchy and inequality. They are: a) the *division of labour* (and power and authority) involved in the production and distribution of goods and services; b) the *pattern of ownership and control of the means or resources* needed for the process; and c) the *representational practices* and *understandings* associated with it.

The production and distribution of goods and services: The international division of labour

As we saw in Chapter 2, Marx's idea that the organisation of material production is the foundation of class has been a staple of sociological explanation. Almost two centuries later, sociologists are generally agreed that the generators of class are more complex. However, in understanding class on a global basis, knowing how the production and distribution of goods and services are organised, and who does what – the *division of labour* – remains central. Despite intensified urbanisation globally (Harvey 2010), almost half of the world's peoples – 3 billion (Food and Agriculture Organization of the United Nations (FAO) 2013) – lives and works mainly, but not exclusively, in rural areas. Around 65 per cent of these are involved in agricultural production that includes agriculture, forestry, fishing and hunting. Most live in Africa, China and South Asia (FAO

2013). Forty per cent of China's workforce, for instance, is employed in agriculture. Their urban-based counterparts, especially in China and the hugely populous countries of South Asia such as India, work mainly in manufacturing, building and construction, and service industry jobs. There are over 1 billion people performing such work in these countries (World Bank 2014b, 2014d).

The vast majority of the workforces in high-income countries, by contrast, no longer produce agricultural or manufactured goods. They provide services in industries that include health care, education, transport, wholesale and retail trade, leisure and recreation, finance and banking, administration and electronic communications. Truck and forklift drivers, teachers, sales assistants, doctors, computer technicians, personal trainers and accountants, for example, are all employed in service industries. Virtually all OECD countries have experienced a steady decline in share of manufacturing in total employment since the 1970s and an absolute decline in the number of manufacturing workers (Pilat et al. 2006). 'Since 1985 the United States has lost an average of 372,000 manufacturing jobs every year' (Moretti 2012: 22). Low and middle-income countries have mounted a formidable challenge to manufacturing in high-income countries, successfully establishing themselves as the main producers of much of the world's manufactured goods. China, for example, is now the world's largest manufacturing nation (UN 2013) especially of mass-produced items such as clothing, footwear, building materials, furniture, household equipment and appliances. More recently, it has begun to move into specialised, high-tech production such as aeronautics, military equipment and pharmaceuticals – traditionally the preserve of high-income countries. Unable to compete with China's lower costs of mass manufacturing, especially in wages for workers, manufacturing in high-income countries has adopted two main strategies. One is to focus on high-tech and 'value added' products requiring 'innovation and development' (Moretti 2012) that involve new jobs and skills, especially related to intellectual and creative work. The manufacture of electronic communications items (such as software) in the United States, for instance, has seen growth in jobs of 562 per cent since the early 1990s (Moretti 2012). Pharmaceuticals, medical equipment and devices (see Chapter 8), motor vehicles (for example, BMW in Germany) and 'luxury goods' (for example, high-priced fashion items by Prada, Gucci, Vuitton, Cartier, Rolex and Burberry) have also accounted for significant expansion. The second strategy adopted by manufacturing in high-income countries is to outsource part or all of their operations to low and middle-income countries, employing local people to do the work at much lower cost than their high-income counterparts (Pilat et al. 2006). Some prestigious European car manufacturers, such as Volvo and Peugeot, have gone down this road, locating most of their production in China. Such an approach, however, obviously limits opportunities for manufacturing employment in high-income countries.

This is not to say that wealthy OECD countries no longer support thriving agricultural industries. Most generate more food than they can sell within their own borders, especially grain, meat and dairy products, in countries such as Australia, Canada, New Zealand and the United States. As a result, many such countries derive substantial income from agricultural exports. They do not employ many people, however, because of large-scale industrialisation of agriculture and intensive factory farming that operates alongside small family farms in which owners and their households are self-employed. By comparison, while more than half of the world's peoples depend on agriculture to survive, they struggle in doing so. India and China, for instance, have been experiencing food deficits while high-income countries have enjoyed rapid growth in food surpluses (FAO 2013). Africa has been especially hard hit by such deficits even though the combination of 'cash crops' (such as coffee, tea, cocoa, nuts, spices, 'feeds', and other raw materials such as cotton) and 'raw foods' (mainly fruit and vegetables) generates an agricultural trade surplus that ends up on international markets (Ng and Aksoy 2008).

The work of producing and distributing goods and services, then, is characterised by a global division of labour whereby most of the workforce in low-income countries, such as those in sub-Saharan Africa and South Asia, are engaged in agricultural subsistence or market production. Those in high-income countries, by comparison, are mainly employed in service industries. Employment in manufacturing and building continues to prevail everywhere, but mostly is concentrated in low and middle-income countries, especially in China. For instance, the city of Shanghai has undergone a government-initiated building and construction program over the past 26 years that has transformed it into a futuristic, high-rise financial and residential metropolis with a population that has more than doubled – now 23 million people – and the world's second-highest skyscraper (Taylor 2013).

The production and distribution of goods and services: The division of labour in the workplace

Regardless of where the production and distribution of goods and services are undertaken internationally, a specific *division of labour* generally characterises the ways in which this process is organised. In the overwhelming majority of situations, the work involved is divided between those who perform the work required and those who manage and control it. In many cases, the work of producing or distributing is sub-divided and the workforce differentiated correspondingly to perform the specific tasks required for each sub-division. In industrialised production, even in high-tech manufacturing, these sub-divisions are often integrated in a 'continuous flow' along an assembly line, as in the production of motor vehicles. Production managers and planners are responsible for 'tasks and decisions... related to equipping and aligning the productive units for a given production process, before the actual assembly can start. This includes setting the system capacity (cycle time, number of stations, station equipment) as well as assigning the work content to productive units (task assignment, sequence of operations)' (Boysen, Fliedner and Scholl 2007: 675). Supervisors are usually employed to oversee the assembly line process and the workers involved according to company guidelines and timelines to deliver 'quality' and 'efficiency'. The sub-division of work can also be organised along the lines of a pyramidal hierarchy, like the civil or public service. The base of the hierarchy comprises the largest 'slice' of the total tasks required, and these are generally regarded as the least complex and difficult – usually routine and repetitive tasks. Ascending the pyramid, the complexity and difficulty of work increase, warranting more skilled and qualified staff who do most of their work with little or no supervision, often exercising independent judgement and providing some guidance and direction to others (Kelly 2002).

Moving higher up the pyramid, the intrinsic complexity and difficulty of work do not intensify but rather give way to a different kind of work – that of middle management. Middle management prevails in most large organisations, in both the corporate and public sectors, and accounts for a large section of the workforce. In Australia, for example, they amount to almost half a million employees (Gleeson 2014). Those engaged in this work are employed to ensure implementation of what their superiors – the senior executives, located at the 'apex' of organisations – determine are the goals of service or goods production and distribution. Middle management engages with and directs workers towards delivering these goals. The executive 'slice' of the pyramid is where most of the planning and strategising occur. What is to be done and by whom – how, where, when, why and with what outcomes – across the organisation is the work of this tier.

While there is a basic division of labour between management and workers, there are further hierarchical differentiations *among* management and *among* workers. Those among workers mainly derive from distinctions accorded the work involved, such as mental versus manual or highly skilled versus routine or unskilled jobs. In hospital workplaces, for example, there are pronounced distinctions between basic service workers – cleaners, meal preparation and delivery staff, building maintenance personnel and so on – and professional health service providers (doctors, nurses and allied health staff) who are, in turn, further differentiated hierarchically (Atwal and Caldwell 2005, Long et al. 2006). Management is divided according to the distinction between the work of planning and strategising, and that associated with directing workers to ensure implementation of plans to achieve goals. These distinctions go hand-in-hand with variations in occupational *recognition*, and the degree of *autonomy* and *control* over one's work and that of others that accompanies them. Those at the bottom of workplace organisation usually experience neither, while executive or senior management enjoy both. Middle managers are also likely to combine autonomy and control in their work but less so than their superiors, precisely because of their accountability to them. Meanwhile, some workers exercise considerable autonomy in what they do in their work and the conditions under which they do so, especially if they are in jobs and occupations that are considered to involve individual skill, judgement and decision-making requiring a university, trade or advanced technical qualification. These workers may even exercise control over others by having to supervise their work on a routine basis.

These distinctions in occupational recognition, and the accompanying distribution of autonomy and control of work associated with the production and distribution of goods and services, operate as major inequalities in the distribution of *symbolic* and *agentic resources*. Intrinsic to the division of labour, then, are significant disparities in the extent to which people can exercise power and authority at work, determining what they do and how, and the conditions under which they do so. Only a very small minority enjoys access to *symbolic* and *agentic* resources associated with work and workplace organisation. Inequality in power and authority in employment is also accompanied by differential access to material resources evident in income disparities. While those in senior management obviously reap the highest rewards, workers 'at the bottom' correspondingly derive the least. Yet, within this broad division there are further hierarchical differentiations of symbolic and agentic resource distribution that correspond with the exercise of power and authority within workplaces.

There are numerous examples of the social dynamic associated with this kind of division of labour in the production and distribution of goods and services. Hospitals, universities, the armed forces, large manufacturing companies, corporate wholesalers, retailers and chain stores illustrate it very well. However, workplaces are not all the same with regard to how they organise work and distribute autonomy and control. Small and medium-sized businesses – usually fewer than 20 employees and mainly in the private sector – are more likely to have what is called 'flat organisation'. In other words, there will be a 'boss', a group of workers and perhaps a supervisor; an arrangement more frequently operating in fast-food chain stores, specialist law and accountancy firms, local specialty shops, small suburban transport companies and specialist manufacturing businesses servicing larger industries, for instance. Nevertheless, the basic division of labour between those who perform work tasks and those who manage and control them prevails, along with the inequality in access to resources that characterises larger organisations. This basic division, in fact, operates as an enduring *structure* or *pattern of practices and relationships* related to goods and services production and distribution, regardless of the size and complexity of the processes involved.

Ownership and control of resources for production and distribution: Global corporations and global division

As the preceding has suggested, most of the world's peoples depend on employment to survive. They are obliged to participate in the production and distribution of goods and services. Yet, the resources needed to enable these processes, such as land, start-up capital, buildings, equipment, expertise and so on, are owned and controlled by a very small minority of people who supply these resources, mainly through *corporations*. From a sociological perspective, corporations are a specific type of significant and enduring social organisation or *institution* (Giddens and Sutton 2014), most of which are owned by the very same people who own and control the resources that corporations use in their production and distribution operations. The large majority of these corporations are based in high-income countries, notably in Europe, North America and parts of Asia/Oceania (principally, Japan, Australia and New Zealand). China, however, has recently emerged as number two, after the United States, among the top 17 countries with the highest number of the world's largest corporations by revenue (Mourdoukoutas 2013). Though the businesses governed by corporations operate throughout the world in diverse places they are often integrated by an overarching corporate management and mission that emanate from their 'home base' or headquarters. Many such businesses are household names globally: for instance, Apple, Nestlé, Shell Oil, BP, ExxonMobil, Toyota, Ford, General Motors, Volkswagen, Hewlett-Packard, Bank of China, Coca-Cola, Samsung, Siemens, Allianz and so on (see Fortune Magazine 2013).

While a key feature of global corporations involves integration, this does not always apply to the relationship between production and distribution, and has implications for the global distribution of ownership of the resources involved in these processes. Though China is the world's largest producer of manufactured goods, for example, owning a sizeable share of the world's resources involved in manufacturing production, the companies involved in this enterprise are not the distributors. The lion's share of China's manufacturing goes to high-income countries, where it is distributed by large retail corporations such as Wal-Mart in the United States, Tesco in the United Kingdom and Coles-Myer in Australia. Wal-Mart is the biggest and richest corporation in the world (Fortune Magazine 2013). Employers and workers in a middle-income country such as China produce the goods while their counterparts in high-income countries distribute them (Harvey 2010). This expansion in distribution in high-income countries has generated increased employment in a wide range of service industries, particularly in retail sales and online shopping, wholesale businesses, transport, haulage and so on. Yet, it is important to acknowledge that the geographic concentration of global corporate investment and management in high-income countries has also spawned significant growth in services such as corporate law, finance and banking, marketing, accountancy and electronic communications.

The international 'über-businesses' of corporate capitalism provide most of the investment needed for production and distribution of goods and services, and receive most of the income generated in the process. This partly explains why sub-Saharan Africa reports an agricultural trade surplus but struggles to supply sufficient food to its peoples. In other words, much of its agricultural land, and the production and distribution generated from it, are owned and run by large, foreign corporations for export to Europe and North America – a situation common among other low-income countries, especially those in South Asia (George 1976, Magdoff and Tokar 2010, McMichael 2010). Such a situation has seen the increasing marginalisation of 'peasant' or subsistence farming in sub-Saharan Africa – a development that, together with the industrialisation of agriculture by foreign corporations, resulted in 2008 in a massive food crisis and the intensification of poverty and hunger (Magdoff and Tokar 2010, Bryceson 2010).

Though based mainly in high-income countries, the world's large corporations have been identified as critical agents of *globalisation*. As British sociologists Anthony Giddens and Phillip Sutton (2014) propose, this refers to the intensification of the links between local events and social relations in one part of the world and what is happening in other parts of the world. The Global Financial Crisis (GFC) that originated in the United States in 2008, for instance, saw a massive diversion of investment by corporations based in wealthy OECD countries away from American and European industry towards a large-scale buy-up of agricultural land and development of industrialised farming in low-income countries, especially in sub-Saharan Africa (Magdoff and Tokar 2010, Bryceson 2010). As explained above, this event played a direct role in triggering a crisis in food and agricultural production for sub-Saharan Africans. It is evident, then, that while globalisation may 'flatten' and integrate the world, as many argue, particularly with respect to electronic communications (see, for example, Friedman 2006), its more significant effects have been to consolidate and deepen *global division* and social inequality (Connell 2007). Not surprisingly, given the evidence outlined so far in this book, the main axis of this division has been between the wealthy OECD countries on the one hand, and the low and middle-income countries on the other, resulting in what many social scientists call the 'Global North' and the 'Global South', respectively (McMichael 2010, Connell 2007). It is evident, then, that the class division created by minority ownership of the resources needed for production and distribution is not confined to nations. It is a global process advanced by corporations and the drive for capital accumulation. However, as the division of labour within workplaces illustrates, such a process is not confined to corporate boardrooms. Workplace division is critical to capital accumulation and the making of class. As the following explains, so, too, is the private ownership and control of wealth and its concentration in the Global North.

Ownership and control of resources for production and distribution: The concentration of wealth in the Global North

The discussion above of the division of labour and hierarchies that prevail in most organisations involved in the production and distribution of goods and services shows how and why one of the most critical of material resources – income – is unequally distributed. It is an intrinsic feature of class. A further key feature of the process involved in the making of class is the private ownership and control of wealth. Like income, wealth distribution both within and between countries is unequal but, by comparison with income inequalities, wealth disparities are astonishingly more pronounced. Patterns of household wealth ownership are one of the commonly used indicators for measuring these disparities.

In 2011, in the United States – the world's largest and richest economy – the top 20 per cent or 'top quintile' of the population owned 84 per cent of all household wealth, while the fourth and fifth quintiles combined (the bottom 40 per cent of the population) owned less than 0.3 per cent (Norton and Ariely 2011: 10–11). The middle quintile weighed in at a little more than 3 per cent. In other words, the majority of Americans – 60 per cent – owned less than 4 per cent of their nation's total household wealth. The concentration of American wealth is illustrated even more starkly by a breakdown in ownership among the members of the 'top decile' or 10 per cent of richest households (Wolff 2009: 2–5, cited in Fireside et al. 2009). Analysis of household wealth in this group shows that the top 1 per cent (first sector) owned 35 per cent of all American wealth, the next 4 per cent (second sector) claimed a further 27 per cent and the next 5 per cent had 11 per cent (third sector): almost 75 per cent of the American 'wealth pie'. The share of the bottom 60 per cent – 4 per cent as mentioned above – is more a sliver than a slice.

Wealth inequality as disclosed by the world's richest country is even more intense on a global basis. As Table 3.2 shows, more than 70 per cent of the world's wealth owned by adults is concentrated among a very small minority – 10 per cent of the global adult population (Davies et al. 2011: 245). The majority of these live in North America, primarily in the United States (22 per cent), Europe (35 per cent) and the wealthy countries of the Asia-Pacific region (including Japan, South Korea, Australia and New Zealand) and several Middle Eastern states (Davies et al. 2011: 237). Only 4 per cent of the richest decile of the world's adults live in Africa and India. This disparity is even greater in relation to the 'top percentile' (1 per cent) of adult wealth ownership: almost 32 per cent of the global total (see Table 3.2). The largest regional group of these hyper-rich are North Americans, as Table 3.2 shows.

The combination of these statistical data shows that there is a marked social division arising from wealth ownership both within countries such as the United States, and between them, as discussed in Chapter 1. A very small minority

TABLE 3.2 *Global wealth shares in 2000 by region, decile and percentile*

REGION	TOP 10%	TOP 1%	ADULT POPULATION (MILLION)	ADULT POPULATION SHARE (%)
World wealth shares (%)	70.7	31.6	–	–
North America	21.7	39.1	225.7	6.1
Latin America & Caribbean	6.5	5.9	302.9	8.2
Europe	35.2	31.4	550.6	14.9
Africa	1.6	1.0	376.3	10.2
China	5.3	0.0	842.1	22.8
India	2.5	0.0	570.6	15.4
Rich Asia-Pacific	21.1	18.9	183.3	5.0
Other Asia-Pacific	6.1	3.8	646.1	17.5
World	100	100	3697.5	100

Source: Adapted from Davies et al. (2011: 245).

owns most of the wealth while the majority's accumulated assets are negligible – usually non-financial assets, such as a home and car (Fireside et al. 2009). What is foundational to this inequality is its source. As the 'Forbes 400 Top Richest Americans', published annually, demonstrates, the overwhelming proportion of wealth derives from ownership of resources that fund the processes of production and distribution of goods and services – in other words, corporate businesses that generate profits, interest and dividends. Table 3.3 provides a selection of some of the individual wealth owners and the sources from which they obtain their wealth from among the richest 400 Americans in the United States in 2013. Many are household names internationally.

Just as a pattern of division and inequality characterises the division of labour and the relations of power and authority in production and distribution of goods and services within and between countries, so, too, is there a distinctive pattern in the ownership of the resources needed to finance the processes involved. As the evidence indicates, this pattern discloses a form of ownership and control of these resources by a remarkably small minority of the global population, and for a very focused purpose – the maximisation of their profits and capital growth. This pattern of ownership and control is one of the most powerful mechanisms by which national and global disparity is generated, making it a central ingredient in the making and re-making of class. Not on its own, of course, as the previous discussion on the division of labour and the relations of power and authority that accompany it, suggest. In fact, the two go

TABLE 3.3 *A selection of the top 400 richest Americans*

BILLIONAIRE RANK	WEALTH SOURCE	BILLIONS (US$)
1. Bill Gates	Microsoft	72.0
6. Christy Walton (& family)	Wal-Mart*	35.4
7. Jim Walton	Wal-Mart*	33.8
8. Alice Walton	Wal-Mart*	33.5
9. S. Robson Walton	Wal-Mart*	33.3
13. Larry Page	Google	24.9
15. Forrest Mars	Confectionary	20.5
19. George Soros	Hedge funds	20.0
20. Mark Zuckerberg	Facebook	19.0
24. Phil Knight	Nike	16.3
30. Rupert Murdoch (& family)	Media	13.4
33. Harold Hamm	Oil and gas	12.4
35. Lauren Powell Jobs	Apple, Disney	11.7
45. Patrick Soon Shiong	Pharmaceuticals	9.0
54. Ralph Lauren	Ralph Lauren	7.7
71. Dennis Washington	Construction, mining	5.8
103. Dianne Hendricks	Roofing	4.4
109. George Lucas	Star Wars	4.2
118. Kirk Kerkorian	Casinos, investments	3.9
134. Donald Trump	TV, real estate	3.5
151. Steven Spielberg	Movies	3.3
161. Mary Dorrance Malone	Campbell Soup	3.1
166. H.F. Johnson	S.C.Johnson & Sons*	3.0
166. I. Johnson	S.C. Johnson & Sons*	3.0
166. S.C. Johnson	S.C. Johnson & Sons*	3.0
166. H. Johnson-Leipold	S.C. Johnson & Sons*	3.0
166. W. Johnson-Marquart	S.C. Johnson & Sons*	3.0
184. Oprah Winfrey	TV	2.9
193. David Rockefeller Snr	Oil, banking	2.8

*Corporate wealth distributed among family members

Source: Compiled from Dolan and Kroll (2013).

hand-in-hand. As we saw in Chapter 2, one of the key processes by which they are connected from a sociological perspective, is *exploitation*. As Marx proposed, the resources-owning-and-controlling minority maintains its superior position by employing the many who do not own or control such resources, paying them a fraction of the market value of what they produce. Central to this story were the two groups or classes created by the process and the relations between them (dominance and subordination) that would be an inevitable and determining feature of everyday life. Though some individuals would move in and out of these groups – upwards or downwards – the division would remain entrenched, with birth into one or the other generally ensuring lifelong assignment to it.

From a 21st-century perspective, Marx's idea of understanding the world as comprised of two warring classes locked into a perpetual struggle of domination and subordination sounds like a story line for science fiction – or *social* science fiction. The Hollywood film *Elysium* (2013), described as 'an American science-fiction, action thriller' in fact portrays an uncannily similar scenario. The main difference, however, is that the wealthy minority of the world escapes to an artificial planet they construct above the Earth, forcing the impoverished masses to remain working in a brutal, post-apocalypse that sustains the minority's extra-terrestrial privilege. In effect, the bourgeoisie and the proletariat morph into utopians and dystopians but there is no mass revolt. Like most Hollywood 'action thrillers', there is an individual hero – the actor Matt Damon. Fortified as a cyborg warrior, he takes on the ruthless forces of darkness – 'CEO'd' by actor Jodie Foster – challenging their entrenchment and heralding a better future for dystopian earthlings. While the Elysium scenario is not immediately imminent, it is evident that global wealth is multiplying in the hands of a very small minority with a corresponding intensification in income inequality in most parts of the world (World Bank 2014e).

Representations and understandings of class

Just as crucial to the making of class as the division of labour and the minority ownership/control of the resources in the production and distribution of goods and services, is the realm of *representations*. These are critical to the social process of symbolisation previously mentioned. 'Representation' is a term that the British-Jamaican sociologist Stuart Hall (1997) developed to refer to all the means we use to express and communicate our thoughts, feelings and understandings, such as speech, writing, visual imagery, dance, fashion and so on. According to Hall, representation is intrinsic to what he called 'signifying practice' – the making and interpreting of meaning. He was strongly influenced by the work of a 20th-century French philosopher, Michel Foucault, who proposed that communication, both written and spoken, is every bit as influential in bringing the world into being as the material things we do, such as the production and distribution of goods and services. Foucault (1980) used the term, 'discourse', to refer to this social process, and argued that it always involved power. Discourses are not simply reflections of reality but makers of it. What is communicated through text – including what is left out – creates the truth of reality for people, shaping their behaviours and actions. Formal knowledges, such as the various branches and modalities of science, are especially powerful discourses, but so, too, are religious and political belief systems. Discourses, in fact, are critical in bringing us into being as individuated *subjects* with specific *identities*. Who we are and what we do is *discursively constructed* rather than the outcome of interior drives and capacities that we develop and act out over time.

Both Foucault and Hall focused their analyses on symbolic practice – of how we make sense of the world and our actions in it, rendering discourse and representation the most critical site of social practice. It is difficult to deny the force of their approach. For example, we cannot make or build things, or do things to, for or with others interpersonally or on a collective basis – as we do daily – without making meaning and drawing on representations and understandings of the world. Such a process is not a *reflection* of 'the real'. It is *constitutive* of it. As such, it plays just as powerful a role in the making of class as the practices of material production and distribution. Together with the division of labour and power/authority in production/distribution, and the ownership/control of the resources needed in the process, it is a structure of practice foundational to the domain of class. How does it work? The short answer is: in complex ways. However, representations and discourses are characterised by a number of specific dynamics. First, they are neither random, nor 'all of a piece'. There are multiple representations or discourses but among these some are *dominant* and others *contestant* or challenging. The former are more pervasive and with greater influence than others in people's understandings of reality. Their dominance is usually linked to dominant *interests* associated with processes of social division, including class (Fairclough 1992). Such interests are usually the major beneficiaries of social division. Often, the power of dominant representations or discourses is illustrated through the extent to which they are not recognised as *social constructions* but, rather, as taken-for-granted 'facts' of everyday life. Dominant discourses or representations are often referred to as *ideology* (Fairclough 1992, Williams 1976).

At the heart of dominant discourse production are powerful institutions or organisations that are central to the operation of a society and whose activities endure over time, such as the media, business and trade union organisations, governments and political parties, and various other instruments of the state, including public sector agencies (see Chapter 7). An especially influential class-based discourse currently propagated by a range of institutions throughout the world is that related to 'free markets' and 'deregulation' – issues addressed more fully in Chapter 7. Widely referred to as *neo-liberalism* (see Chapter 7), this discourse asserts – over and over, and with limited opposition – that everybody's interests, usually expressed in terms of 'the nation', depends on the success of business and the right of markets to be the main producers and distributors of everything wherever possible; that is, wherever profits can be made. Yet, it is evident from the data on socio-economic inequality and health disparities both within and between countries, as illustrated in this chapter, that global production and distribution based on markets and capital accumulation do not advance everybody's interests equally. In fact, as we have seen, such inequalities remain as entrenched as ever, with minority ownership of productive resources becoming ever more concentrated. The discourse of neo-liberalism actively contributes to the making of class because it advances the interests of the dominant class by proposing that they are everybody's interests when the evidence shows they are not. Such a discourse is a good example of ideology. It obscures the social dynamics of class, leaving unchallenged understandings of socio-economic inequalities and health inequities as the outcome of individual advantage or disadvantage, and fortune or misfortune.

How class gets into people's bodies as health and illness

This chapter has one last task: to address the question of how the social process of class gets into people's bodies as health and illness. There is, after all, enormous bodily diversity. We all come with deoxyribonucleic acid, or DNA, that encodes us as individually unique. Yet, our DNA also binds us together as humans distinct from other organisms. DNA is made of chemical bases,

99 per cent of which are the same in all people (Calladine et al. 2004). It is how these bases are configured or sequenced, and how they interact with certain molecular dynamics, that distinguishes each of us biologically at birth and in our development over time. This individual genetic heritage is one of the biological dimensions involved in people's health fortunes but, as genetic science demonstrates, genes associated with adult illnesses are 'non-deterministic'. 'Particular clusters or networks of genes result in greater or lesser "predispositions" to various illnesses, but the actual consequences of these predispositions for the organism will depend upon its environment and experiences' (Evans, Hodge and Pless 1994: 178). More significantly, in terms of understanding how the social – in this case class dynamics – gets into people's bodies as health and illness, it is our common physiological inheritance as a human species that is more critical than individual gene profiles. Though there is still much more to learn about how this works because of the complexity involved, the bioscientific evidence is conclusive: the health effects of environment and experiences associated with class, in fact, depend on 'biological pathways' that we share as human beings (Evans 1994). What are these and how are they connected to the social dynamics and unequal access to key social resources associated with health inequities discussed in this chapter?

As our earlier evidence on SES and health disparities shows, social hierarchy, division and competition among people generate increasingly worse health outcomes as we proceed 'down the ladder', and incrementally better ones as we ascend it. This hierarchy derives from one of the central dynamics of class: a division of labour that exists primarily to maximise the production and distribution of goods and services. In order to achieve this goal, there is a chain of command and control, with those at the top wielding most of it and those at the bottom having little or none. This hierarchy of control is not confined to workplaces. It translates into unequal access to material, symbolic and agentic resources in people's everyday lives, as demonstrated by the disparities in people's incomes and education, and the correspondingly differential *struggles* people face in obtaining housing, a healthy diet, clothing, transport, education for their children, restorative recreation and physical activity. As significant are the concomitantly differentiated barriers to, and opportunities for, participating in activities that bring recognition of people's worth as individuals and a sense of being able to act on and influence the directions and outcomes of one's life.

Psychoneuroimmunological (PNI) research, studies in 'brain plasticity' (Kolb and Gibb 2011), and investigation of the physiological responses to stress of primates – both human and non-human – reveal compelling findings about the biology and embodiment of social division and competition. At the heart of much of this work is the relationship between stress, the 'fight-or-flight' response, and cortisol – a hormone released by the adrenal gland when a threat to survival or well-being is seen, heard or sensed in some way. In short, exposure to stress turns on the fight-or-flight response, which releases cortisol into the blood in order to enhance the ability to deal with the perceived threat. Sweating and increased heart rate are overt bodily signs of the reaction but there are also 'micro-level' responses associated with stimulating or dampening the immune system. Regular triggering of this process, especially when it results in failure to prevent or constrain its effects, produces tissue damage and 'greater risk of future injury or deterioration' (Evans, Hodge and Pless 1994: 170). Known health consequences are depression and anxiety, high blood pressure, ischaemic heart disease, premature ageing and death, and, among children, a diminished capacity to learn and develop emotionally because of neuronal damage (McEwen 2008a, Kolb and Gibb 2011).

More recently, commentary by two renowned genetic researchers, published in the most reputable scientific journal in the world, *Nature*, explains that ongoing psychological stress and the release of cortisol 'shorten genetic telomeres'. This process produces a wide range of severely damaging health outcomes, especially among children (Blackburn and Epel 2012), as explained in the box.

Cameron Diaz, stress and telomeres

The American actor Cameron Diaz is used to playing many different characters, often glamorous and seductive. As genetic researchers Elizabeth Blackburn and Elissa Epel noted recently, Diaz's 2006 film, *The Holiday*, showed her in the shoes of a woman whose life was spinning out of control, and exclaiming, 'Severe stress...causes the DNA in our cells to shrink until they can no longer replicate. So when we're stressed we look haggard' (cited in Balckburn and Epel 2012: 169).

As the scientists remarked, 'Hollywood got that science right. The DNA to which Diaz's character alludes is the segment that makes up telomeres, structures that cap and protect the ends of chromosomes. She was referring to our 2004 publication – the first to link chronic psychological stress to compromised telomere maintenance' (Blackburn and Epel 2012: 169).

As they then went on to explain, subsequent research has consistently disclosed that chronic stress in a variety of forms is linked to – and most likely causes – shorter telomeres. At the same time, telomere shortness and stress have strong associations with common conditions such as cardiovascular diseases and diabetes. These connections are so pervasive and consistent that the message is clear: in the absence of alleviation of severe stress arising from the relentlessness of sustained threats in people's lives such as war, financial hardship, abuse and emotional neglect, particularly in children, there will be 'exponentially higher costs further down the line – personal, economic and otherwise' (Blackburn and Epel 2012: 169).

As the editors of a 2012 issue of *Nature* commented:

> Now, biologists are starting to render visible how one aspect of the environment – stress – leaves marks on the body . . . [I]t is most potent when it occurs during brain development, a surprisingly long period of time stretching from the third trimester of pregnancy to the end of adolescence. These stress-induced changes increase vulnerability to all sorts of conditions, including psychiatric disorders and antisocial behaviour. (*Nature*, Editorial 2012: 149)

Conclusions

It is evident from the research on the biological pathways of stress and control that living with prolonged stress – both in workplaces and beyond – is one of the critical mechanisms by which class dynamics get into people's bodies. The illustrations of this bio-social process have focused on those who bear the greatest health damage associated with it – those with more limited access to social resources and control over their lives. Yet, it is clear that this damage is the product of a relationship of social division and power in which there are also health beneficiaries. They experience greater control and less stress in their lives because of their superior location in the division of labour and/or their ownership and control of resources, associated with the production and distribution of goods and services. As demonstrated by the astonishing disparities in wealth and income internationally, it is apparent that social division and competition for survival are even more dramatic and devastating in most low and middle-income countries. Class dynamics associated with capital accumulation are truly globalised and globalising, and with them, the socio-economic inequalities that are now so well documented by global agencies such as the World Bank and the WHO. Health inequities associated with SES, then, are not simply the products of various combinations of social factors related to how we live and work across the globe. Rather, they are the embodied outcome of a specific domain of social relations and dynamics that operates on an extraordinary scale and with remarkable relentlessness. The dynamics of class inevitably generate social division – both nationally and globally – and with it a process that advantages a very small minority at the expense of the very large majority. These dynamics and the health dimensions that accompany them are certainly pernicious. Yet, as the following chapters show, class is not the only social domain responsible for the consistent production of unnecessary adversity and the health costs it imposes both within and between countries.

Questions for discussion

1 What is the social health gradient? How can we tell it exists in relation to mortality and life expectancy both within and between countries?

2 What are the main resources necessary for health from a sociological perspective? How does access to these resources affect health?

3 What distinguishes class from other social processes involved in producing social inequalities and health disparities? What are the main structures of practice that comprise it?

4 How does the international division of labour in producing and distributing goods and services produce class division?

5 What are the main purposes of the workplace division of labour? How does it contribute to the making of class?

6 How does corporate ownership and control of resources for production and distribution produce class divisions both within and between countries? In what sense are corporations critical agents of globalisation and global division?

7 How does the concentration of global wealth in the Global North contribute to the production of class? How does it contribute towards health disparity?

8 What does it mean to say that representations and understandings of class are just as significant in the making of class as the practices of material production and distribution?

9 How does class get into people's bodies as health and illness?

4 Gender and health

Overview

- What distinguishes gender from other processes of social division? What does it mean to say that gender dynamics are historically and socially variable?

- How does a sex-differences approach to health characterise the health of men and women? What are the limitations of this approach?

- What is a gender order and what does it mean to say that it is patriarchal?

- What evidence is there to say that gender inequality prevails on a global scale?

- What is gendered health? What are examples of gender dynamics involved in it?

- What is the relationship between gender dynamics, intersectionality and health disparity?

- How are gender inequality and patriarchy evident in health disparity?

China 1911

'My grandmother's feet had been bound when she was two years old. Her mother...first wound a piece of white cloth about twenty feet long round her feet, bending all the toes except the big toe inward and under the sole. Then she placed a large stone on top to crush the arch' (Chang 1991:31). As Jung Chang (1991: 31–2) recounts in her acclaimed personal history about her life in China, the pain from footbinding had been so agonising that her grandmother had screamed in agony, fainting over and over. The procedure had been repeated over several years, with the feet bound day and night to stop them from recovering. Though there had been no reprieve from the pain throughout the process and Jung's grandmother had pleaded with her mother to stop, the mother could only weep, telling her daughter her life would be ruined without bound feet and that her future happiness depended on it. As Jung explains, such a practice had prevailed in China for about a thousand years. It was only in bed at night that the binding could be relaxed – rarely ever removed and rarely ever witnessed by men. Removal of the binding usually revealed rotting, stinking flesh.

Though a former practice confined to China, the gruesome torture of binding the feet of young girls illustrates a virtually universal phenomenon. It is the practice of making visible the *sexual reproductive distinction* (Connell 2009) between human beings. While this distinction is biological, making it visible is quintessentially a social act. By comparison with footbinding in China, however, most other social methods of making visible sexual difference in childhood – apart from genital mutilation – have been far less physically deforming. Not that footbinding was practised explicitly to torture and cripple young girls. It was designed and conducted ostensibly to enhance young women's marital prospects, conveying both feminine respectability and sexual attractiveness (Chang 1991: 32). Elsewhere in the world, and at other times in human history, the practice of marking the sexual reproductive distinction on children's bodies has been consistently related to the futures that children were imagined and expected to live. In the 'developed' world of Europe, this practice usually involved dress and adornment. For example, while 16th and 17th-century portraits of the children of European nobility depict what look like miniature versions of their adult counterparts, they capture in fine detail the distinctions that render the subjects unmistakably girls or boys, and future noblewomen and men.

Spain 1600s

A famous painting (*Las Meninas*, Spanish for The Maids of Honour) by Spanish artist Diego Velázquez foregrounds the young aristocratic child, Margarita of Austria, by portraying her in the dress and bearing of adult women who were being painted around the same time (Portus et al. 2004: 217, 347). Similarly, Velázquez's painting of the six-year-old 'Prince Baltasar Carlos as a Hunter' (1635–36) represents this young boy as a young noble*man* in the making. The prince poses with precocious aplomb, magisterially occupying the lands of a royal estate while dressed in hunting garb, armed with a gun and flanked by hunting dogs poised to obey their young master's commands (Portus et al. 2004).

Gender as a specific domain of social practice

Representation from the portraiture of early modern Europe and the now-defunct practice of Chinese footbinding are both features of a social process that plays a central role in the making of social inequality and health inequity – *gender*. It is nonetheless distinguished from class and other domains of divisive social practice that result in health disparity, namely indigeneity, ethnicity and the state (see Chapters 5, 6 and 7). *What makes gender so specific in its relationship to social inequality is that it concentrates on the sexual reproductive distinction among human beings and makes it matter in terms of people's access to material, symbolic and agentic resources.* It actually produces 'girls' and 'boys', 'women' and 'men', making the biological sex difference between them a key determinant of who gets to do what, when, how, why, with whom and with what consequences in everyday life. In the process, it confers greater benefits upon men, both within and between countries, and so it inextricably involves the exercise of *power*. Not that all men benefit to the same degree and in the same ways. Gender interacts with other processes of social division, such as class. In fact, one of the defining features of all such dynamics is that they mix and merge with each other – a phenomenon some sociologists call *intersectionality* (see Chapter 6).

Gender does not operate like a conveyor belt that churns out two variations of a basic model of the human. Rather, it produces social mixtures whereby in some circumstances, some groups of women will be more advantaged than some groups of men *and* other women in terms of access to social resources. In most of the wealthy OECD countries of the world, for instance, young women from middle and upper-class families are more likely to gain entry to university based legal and medical education than young women *and* young men from working-class families. Gender, then, does not work in such a way that it systematically advantages *all* men at the expense of *all* women, *all* of the time, as discussed further below. Nevertheless, it is common for an *aggregate,* or broad pattern, of social inequality to be produced by gender dynamics across a range of sites or settings, from organisations and institutions such as the family, corporations and public sector agencies, to whole societies and, indeed, across the globe.

The distinctiveness of gender is produced by a *combination* of what Raewyn Connell (2009: 73) has described as *structures of gendered relations and practices.* As she has commented, however, these do not always make the reproductive difference a basis for division and conflict. Gender processes can establish relations of cooperation, solidarity and even affection and love among human beings. Yet, the usual pattern involves mobilising sex difference to exercise power over another, including through abuse and violence. So, like class, gender is a complex social dynamic that, also like class, encompasses various structures of practice. Gender dynamics develop in a variety of ways, subject to time and place, and are not intrinsically or necessarily hierarchical. In this chapter, however, our discussion of gender focuses on explaining how it operates in relation to social inequality and health disparity.

Gender, sex differences and health

The dominant approach to gender and health throughout the world is one that focuses on *sex differences* (male/female) and measurable health outcomes of the kind outlined in previous chapters. In aggregate, the picture portrayed by the statistical patterns used in the process suggests that women live longer, sicker lives than men. Men, on the other hand, live shorter lives characterised by more injury and substance use problems, mainly tobacco and alcohol but also illicit drugs.

The World Bank's recent 'development indicators' on global male and female mortality rates by country, for example, document the widely reported 'fact' of women's greater longevity as measured by medical and epidemiological research (Waldron 1967, Eskes and Haanen 2007, Ginter and Simko 2013). According to these indicators, the global mortality rate in 2013 for the period 2007–12 for men aged 15 to 60 years was 194 for every 1000 men and 138 for every 1000 women in the same age range (World Bank 2014c). These figures mean that if you are a man aged between 15 and 60 years, the probability of you dying between these ages is 194 in 1000, while a woman's chances in the same age range are 138 in 1000. Clearly, your chances of longevity are increased by being 'female'. A similar approach is evident in relation to rates of morbidity collated by epidemiologists. Summarising this data in relation to 'industrialized nations', American sociologist Chloe Bird and colleagues (2012: 146) reported the following:

> [M]en develop more life-threatening conditions (for example, cancer and cardiovascular disease) at younger ages than do women. In contrast, women have higher rates of chronic debilitating disorders such as autoimmune diseases and rheumatoid disorders, as well as irritating but less life-threatening diseases such as anaemia, arthritis, migraines and thyroid diseases…
> [W]omen experience more physical illness, sick days and hospitalizations than men (even excluding reproductive related care)…

At the same time, women's rates of mental and emotional morbidity, based on measures of mental disorders and diseases, are consistently identified as exceeding those of men. The WHO (2009a), for instance, has reported that, *worldwide*, anxiety and depression are significantly more common among women, who are also more likely to seek treatment for such conditions than men.

Sex differences in injury statistics throughout the world, however, consistently reveal higher rates among men. According to the WHO (2013f), motor vehicle accidents are one of the main sources of this difference:

From a young age, males are more likely to be involved in road traffic crashes than females. More than three-quarters (77%) of all road traffic deaths occur among men. Among young drivers, young males under the age of 25 years are almost 3 times as likely to be killed in a car crash as young females.

Yet, there are also other major sources. On a global basis, men incur significantly higher rates of workplace injuries (Schofield 2014, Courtenay 2011) and injuries from violence (homicide and suicide) (Schofield 2012a, Courtenay 2011). WHO (2010b: 11–12) global data indicate that men's rates of death from violent injuries are around twice those of women. While their rates of mental disorders and diseases are lower than those of women, as outlined above, their damaging consumption of alcohol and use of tobacco and illicit drugs greatly exceed women's (WHO 2005a, WHO 2010c, Greaves 2007, Courtenay 2011, Busfield 2012, Schofield 2012a).

Based on the combined evidence related to sex differences and health outcomes, many conclude that gender operates in such a way that it causes poor health among *both* men and women but in *distinctive* ways – same but different. As a consequence, men as a sex are no more disadvantaged in relation to their health than women and vice versa. The sex-differences-in-health approach, both nationally and internationally, basically suggests there is no gender disparity in health. Rather, men and women have 'gender-specific' health needs that policy and health services should address equally (Schofield 2004). The Australian government, for example, proclaims a commitment to both a 'National Male Health Policy' and a 'National Women's Health Policy'. The United States government professes a similar approach but does not have formalised, gender-specific policies. There are, however, 'facts' that raise significant doubts about 'the facts' of sex-differentiated health outcomes.

Closer examination of the World Bank's global development indicators on sex-differentiated mortality by country, for example, does not reveal universally better outcomes for women. If you are female and live in Botswana, for example, your chances of a long life are considerably more diminished than the average for men globally (see above). The probability of death for women in Botswana between the ages of 15 and 60 years is 738 in 1000 (World Bank 2014c)! Not that Botswana is unique among sub-Saharan African countries in terms of women's mortality rate. If you are a woman born in virtually any sub-Saharan country, the 'average global man' will likely outlive you – and by a considerable number of years. The dramatically increased probability of death among these women is even more pronounced by comparison with men in Qatar in the Middle East, where the male adult mortality rate is 65 in 1000. The World Bank's sex-differentiated adult mortality rates for all of the countries of the world in fact reveal remarkable variations in men's and women's chances of dying before age 60. So much so that it is simply not true to say that women live longer than men or that men die earlier, *unless* we are talking about a statistical construction that asks us to believe that men and women are *two distinct categories* of human beings based on reproductive difference. As the following explains, the *social* realities of life mean that sex difference per se exerts very limited impact on health (Schofield et al. 2000). As significantly, the explanatory framework built around it – a sex-differences approach – does not account for the complexities actually operating in the gendering of health and the disparities associated with it.

Gender as biological and social categories

A sex-differences approach to gender tells a 'two-realms' story, and informs prevailing understandings of gender the world over. From this perspective, women and men are *static categories* of human beings, distinguished by reproductive sexual characteristics that go hand-in-hand with sex-differentiated (and differentiating) 'socialisation', or upbringing. Gender differences arise from a combination of *both* biology – sometimes called 'nature' – and sex roles – sometimes called 'nurture'. The result is so polarising, some suggest, that men may as well be from Mars and women from Venus. From the sex-differences viewpoint, human beings are understood to be characterised by a 'body dimorphism' (Connell 2009: 59) upon which social difference, or gender, is elaborated. Choice of clothing and differentiated colour schemes for babies, toddlers and children (usually pink for girls and blue for boys), for instance, illustrates the process and how it begins from the very outset of people's lives. Yet, there are critical aspects of this two-realms story that do not add up. As Raewyn Connell (2009: 59) put it, 'human bodies are dimorphic only in limited ways', and human behaviour far exceeds any kind of dimorphism, as the following account of her explanation shows.

Gender b[l]ending

Physical differences between males and females do not remain unchanged over the course of their lives. Among infants and young children, male and female bodies are almost the same. There are negligible differences 'between a two-year old girl and a two-year old boy. Even the obviously different external reproductive organs – penis, clitoris, scrotum and labia – develop embryonically from a common starting point' (Connell 2009: 52). Old age actually makes male and female bodies more similar, especially in relation to hormonal balance.

Even as young adults, Connell observes, males as a group and females as a group share many physical features. Adult females are on average a little shorter than adult males, but within each group there is considerable variation with respect to the average difference. A very large number of individual women are taller than individual men. Yet, due to social custom, we tend not to notice this physical fact (Connell 2009: 52).

Brain anatomy and function are more complex examples of gender overlap. Differences between women and men have been identified in relation to use of particular areas of the brain in language processing (Connell 2009). But, as the neuroscientist Lesley Rogers (2000: 34) explains: 'The brain does not choose neatly to be either a female or a male type. In any aspect of brain function that we can measure there is considerable overlap between females and males' (see also Rogers 2010).

Turning to the sex-role dimension, 'human behaviour is hardly dimorphic at all, even in areas related to sexual reproduction. For instance, while few men do child care with infants, it is also true that, at any given time, most women are not doing this work either' (Connell 2009: 59).

As significantly, as Connell (2009) recounted, there is now a solid body of psychological research demonstrating that, far from what popular – or stereo-typical – accounts insist, women and men are *not* dichotomised along lines of character: emotional, intuitive, nurturant *versus* rational, aggressive, pro-miscuous, for instance (see also Wester et al. 2002, Hyde 2005). Nor are there any other gender dichotomies with respect to general intelligence, cognitive skills, self-esteem, suggestibility, achievement motivation, and auditory and visual abilities, to name a few from a very long list (Archer and Lloyd 1982, Hyde 2005). Among the statistically measurable psychological differences between men and women, close to 80 per cent are 'small or close to zero' (Hyde 2005: 586). Clearly, while psychological differences do exist between men and women, the magnitude of such differences does not support *polarising* sex stereotypes. Men and women are psychologically more similar than they are different.

Gender inequality and patriarchy

Despite the absence of significant biological and psychological differences between the sexes, patterns of gender division are widespread. The pervasiveness of this pattern throughout the world indicates a specific kind of global *gender order* (Connell 2009) – one that is profoundly unequal and patriarchal. These are processes of gender division that are characterised by control and exploitation of women, and that return a significantly greater dividend to men as a group (Connell 2009). The patriarchal dividend has an inverse relationship to gender equality: it declines as gender equality grows. An example is the institution of patriarchal marriage or 'intimate partnership', found all over the world. Patriarchal marriages and intimate partnerships are personal relationships in which the male partner gains greater access to valued social resources such as income, housing, social status and respect, emotional support and the opportunity to control and influence his life at the expense of his female partner. The costs to women partners are generally exacted through the routine expectations and practices of these relationships. One of the most common of these is women's responsibility for all or most of the unpaid work of maintaining households and caring for children. Yet, there are many others, including the lack of financial independence associated with resistance or hostility by male partners to women's employment, and violence and abuse (physical, sexual and emotional) by male partners. The latter also often encompasses economic violence associated with control of the income women earn if they are allowed or forced to do paid work (United Nations 2010).

The benefits of gender inequality to various groups of men are especially well illustrated in relation to business and political life. As we saw in Chapter 3, *Forbes* magazine's '400 Richest People in America' in 2013 lists only a very small number of women. *Fortune* magazine's annual list of the 'top' 500 giant global companies in 2013 shows that only 23 of these had a woman CEO, or 4.6 per cent of the total 'top' positions. In other words, men amounted to 95.4 per cent of corporate bosses, reaping the lion's share of the rewards associated with these positions.

In political life, men also lead the way in hugely larger numbers than women, again enjoying a much greater proportion of the benefits that accrue from such participation. According to the World Bank (2014a), women held 22 per cent of the combined number of seats in all of the world's parliaments in 2013. There were marked variations internationally, with women holding less than

10 per cent of parliamentary seats in many low-income countries, such as Egypt, Iran, Lebanon, Myanmar, Sri Lanka, Congo Republic, Nigeria, Swaziland, Papua New Guinea, Solomon Islands and Tonga. In high-income European countries (notably Finland, Norway, Sweden, Denmark, Iceland, the Netherlands and Belgium) there was approximate gender parity, with women holding 38–50 per cent of parliamentary seats across the board. Yet, high national income was not a prerequisite for parliamentary seats held, as the percentages of seats held by women in the following countries demonstrate: Rwanda (64 per cent), Cuba (49 per cent), Seychelles (44 per cent), Senegal (43 per cent), South Africa (42 per cent), Nicaragua (40 per cent), Mozambique (39 per cent) and Timor-Leste (39 per cent). High national income, in fact, disclosed no guarantee of a gender balance in the occupation of parliamentary seats, as the percentages held by women in the Anglo-democracies of Australia (26 per cent), Canada (25 per cent), the United Kingdom (23 per cent) and the United States (18 per cent) showed. The differences in the average proportions of parliamentary seats held by women on a global basis, then, were quite small. The proportion in low-income countries was 21 per cent; 20 per cent in middle-income countries and 25 per cent in high-income countries. All of which is to suggest that, apart from a comparative few notable exceptions (that is, fewer than 20 countries), men basically run the show when it comes to key political institutions, such as parliamentary decision-making (see Chapter 7), and they do so on a global basis.

Further, recent World Bank (2014a) data on men's and women's participation in other influential, senior decision-making positions, such as senior public sector officials and managers, suggest a similar but nonetheless varied picture – at least in countries that have collected such information. Women are reported to comprise from 3 per cent of these positions in Pakistan to as much as 55 per cent in the Philippines. In the rich democracies, women occupy on average 33–40 per cent of these positions.

Both within and between countries, then, the reproductive distinction is made to matter in terms of who gets to do the influential, prestigious and highly rewarded work of running global businesses and political institutions that establish the broad conditions of our lives. But its effects far exceed the realm of elite decision-making and global power. Reproductive difference is mobilised in the organisation of routine employment, its conditions and remuneration, affecting most of the world's peoples in generally divisive ways – and on a daily basis. Overall, in 2012, 51 per cent of all women aged 15 years or over, compared with 77 per cent of men in this age range, were engaged in paid work. Women accounted for only 40 per cent of the entire global workforce

(World Bank 2014b). Women's rate of participation varied greatly by global region, with the lowest occurring in North Africa and the Middle East – where women comprised 21 per cent of the labour force on average – and the highest, at 45 per cent, in both sub-Saharan Africa and the high-income countries of Europe. Women were much more likely than men to be employed part-time, performing on average around two-thirds of all recorded global, part-time employment (World Bank 2014d). The types of jobs they did were also generally less well paid, but this varied globally according to the sectors in which they were employed. In the world's poorest region of South Asia, between 2009 and 2012, employment in the worst paid industry – agricultural work – accounted for 59 per cent of the total of women's labour-force participation in that region (World Bank 2014d). For men in this region, it comprised 46 per cent of their employment. Women in wealthy countries, such as the Anglo-democracies and those in the European Union, by contrast, were concentrated in service-industry jobs. Eighty-six per cent of all women's employment in these countries was located in this sector (World Bank 2014d), with opportunities for markedly higher income than that offered in agriculture.

In the light of this gendered pattern of employment participation and elite decision-making, the income disparity between men and women on a global basis is hardly surprising. Some estimate that, worldwide, men's share of all income is not quite double that of women's but not too far from it, at 80 per cent more (Connell 2009). According to the United Nation's most recent 'World's Women' report, based on International Labour Office (ILO) analyses of wage trends and excluding all other kinds of income, a 'gender pay gap exists everywhere' (United Nations 2010: 97).

'A gender pay gap exists everywhere'

The 'World's Women' reports that 'women's wages represent between 70 and 90 per cent of men's wages in a majority of countries' (United Nations 2010: 97). The gap is smaller for Europe, where recent estimates for 30 countries disclose a variation of 15 to 25 per cent.

By comparison, 'women in the Republic of Korea earn 68 per cent of what men earn. In Brazil and the United Kingdom there are a few occupations in which women earn more than men: 5 out of 31 occupations in the former and 8 out of 116 in the latter. In most occupations in these two countries, women earn from 60 to 100 per cent of what men earn' (United Nations 2010: 97). Where the ratio of women's average earnings to men's average earnings is expressed per 100, women's average earnings ratio in Australia is 88 across all occupations – 12 per cent lower than gender parity.

The ILO reports that this pay gap has narrowed over the past five years in many countries, but this is mainly attributable to a contraction in men's employment rather than an improvement in women's labour market participation and their remuneration (ILO Global Wage Report 2013a). The decline in men's employment is largely attributable to the 'Global Financial Crisis' (GFC), which originated in the United States in 2008. Unequal earnings between men and women are closely associated with a further dimension of gender relations, whereby sex difference is socially operationalised in determining who gets to do the work involved and what financial reward and social recognition accrue to it. This is the realm of domestic work that, according to the international System of National Accounts that defines productive activity and calculates its economic value (cited in United Nations 2010: 98), includes 'food preparation, dish washing, cleaning and upkeep of dwelling, laundry, ironing, handicraft, gardening, caring for pets, construction and repairs, shopping, installation, servicing and repair of personal and household goods, childcare, care of sick, elderly or disabled household members, etc.' Domestic work is considered to be outside the 'productive boundary' and, therefore, 'counts for nothing' (Waring 1988) in economic terms. Though men may be more likely to take responsibility for some of these tasks, such as construction and repairs, women everywhere do most of the others, as women's time spent on domestic work illustrated in Figure 4.1 shows. Preparing meals, cleaning, caring for household members and shopping account for most of women's time spent on domestic work (United Nations 2010: 101).

Gendered health

Despite the depth and breadth of the disparities between men and women on a global basis, gender dynamics do not always operate patriarchally or produce outright division and inequality between men and women, and among them. Sometimes they produce no hierarchy. Studies of gender dynamics in Australian organisations, such as public policymaking units and the governing boards of Olympic sports, have shown how men and women in some of the sites investigated established relations and procedures of gender equality in managing and performing their activities (Schofield and Goodwin 2005, Adriaanse and Schofield 2013). Men and women worked cooperatively and enjoyably with each other in roughly equal numbers and at all levels of the process, in the absence of animosity, rivalry and sexist 'put downs', and with a commitment to advancing gender equality. Legislation passed in the Nordic

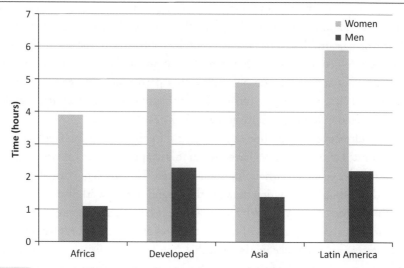

FIGURE 4.1 *Time spent on domestic work (hours per day) by region and sex, 1999–2008 (latest available)*
Source: United Nations 2010: 100.

countries, such as Norway in 1981 (the Gender Equality Act), has also result-ed in a marked decline in men's dominance, not only on publicly appointed boards, councils and committees but also on boards of publicly owned en-terprises and large joint stock companies in the private sector. The Act and its amendments in the 2000s mandated at least 40 per cent representation by women in these organisations. As these illustrations show, the operation of power in gender dynamics is not monolithic. It does not usually operate as a force that bears down upon and trammels everything and everybody within its wake. It is resisted and contested by countervailing responses and reac-tions. The variability in how gendered power works is expressed in the con-cept of *gender regimes* (Connell 2009). In other words, the relations between men and women, and among them, can be configured in various ways, from total subjugation of women by men, to equality, involving cooperation and solidarity between them. Yet, as previously mentioned, the dominant configu-ration across the globe and within countries – the gender order – is one of male dominance and gender inequality.

Yet, however gender relations are organised and enacted, they rarely, if ever, work in isolation from class and other social divisions such as those associat-ed with ethnicity, indigeneity and the state (see Chapters 5, 6 and 7). These *intersections* – or mixing and merging processes – mean that some groups of men face a lot more health trouble than other men; and some groups of women have worse health than other women. But, by contrast with the sex-differences approach to gender and health, a gender-relations-and-intersections perspective does not see all men on one side with a particular, aggregate pattern of health and all women on the other with a different one. How then *does* gender work in relation to men's health and women's health?

In addressing this question, we return to the epidemiological 'fact' of men's greater rates of injury. As we have seen in this chapter and the previous, workplace injuries occur overwhelmingly among men. The problem is usually represented as a simple correlation between the magnitudes of workplace injury and death, and the category, 'men by occupation'. It is often accompanied by a further statistical correspondence between the rates of women's workplace injuries and deaths, and their occupational profile. Yet, looking a little more closely at the data on men's employment injuries by occupation, it is evident that there are marked differences *among* men. Those employed in traditional blue-collar jobs carry the greatest burden of workplace injuries (and/or deaths) by comparison with their white-collar counterparts in professional, administrative and managerial jobs (see, for example, Draper, Turrell and Oldenburg 2004). This disparity among men arises largely as a result of the class-based organisation of employment that men continue to dominate (Collinson and Hearn 2009) despite increased workforce participation by women since the 1960s. Working-class men incur a disproportionate rate of workplace injury because they dominate participation in the most injurious areas of employment, such as mining, building and construction, transportation and storage, agriculture, forestry and fishing, and heavy manufacturing (Schofield, Reeve and McCallum 2014). Their dominance, however, is also gendered insofar as they rarely work alongside women who could be their girlfriends, partners, wives, sisters, mothers or daughters – in other words, working-class women. This is because working-class employment has developed through a gendered social process. The incorporation of the reproductive distinction between bodies has been critical in the organisation of work.

Being reproductively female or male has played a determining role in differential access to the labour market, occupational location, workplace conditions and rates of pay. Working-class men historically have tended to occupy more of the available jobs, especially full-time jobs, and have participated across a wider range of occupations than their female counterparts. Their greater and more diverse employment has yielded them more material benefits but has also exposed them at significantly higher rates to injurious and fatal work. In the high-income countries at least, the factor that has most influenced this outcome has been adoption by both management and trade unions of aggressive exclusion of women in hazardous jobs since the 19th century. In the United Kingdom, for instance, the 'coal mining industry was several hundred years old by the nineteenth century' (Bartrip and Burman 1983: 13), and men, women and children were all recruited to work in it when the Factory Acts prevented women and their children from competing with men for access to those jobs. This gendering of employment has seen a thoroughgoing *masculinisation* of such work and men's bodily damage in doing it. With global division and the international division of labour, much of this injury has been exported to the working-class men of the Global South (Schofield 2014).

Gendering in employment and economic life, however, is not simply confined to the organisational division of labour. It also involves the way in which the social processes of enacting this organisation renders workers distinctively *masculine* or *feminine*, and how they relate to each other as men and women. This is basically what gender regimes are about. Gendering and sexual difference in workplaces operate emotionally and symbolically, and are as central in the making of people's identities and workplace relationships as they are to the division of labour. Relationships and activities at work are a social mechanism by which people bring themselves into being as particular kinds of gendered people. A notable feature of this process historically is the relentlessness with which men have sought to *segregate* themselves from women in employment, frequently expressing their collective separateness in hostile and sometimes violent treatment of women. The aggressive harassment and exclusion by mining workers of women who have attempted to work side by side with men in mines in Australia, Canada and the United States, for example, illustrates the intensity of this separatism (Moore 1996, Pini and Mayes 2008). They also disclose a *gender regime* of patriarchal dominance. Maintaining sexual segregation in the workplace has been critical to many forms of working-class masculine identity, but no more so than for men in more privileged workplace situations such as management and highly paid professions, where men have also predominated through women's exclusion (Connell 2011). Until comparatively recently, legal, medical and other professional occupations have been male-dominated, deriving substantial material and symbolic dividends as a result (see Chapter 8 in relation to the medical profession, for example).

Men's greater rates of injuries from violence, as indicated by higher mortality associated with suicide and homicide, also illustrate the operation of a complex gendered dynamic and its connection with the making of masculine identity (Jaworski 2014, Morrell 2001, Connell 1995). So, too, do men's rates of injury from road traffic accidents (Walker, Butland and Connell 2000). Certainly men's more intensive development and use of skills in exercising aggression and physical force are expressed in their greater violence-related injury; while their higher rates of ownership of motor vehicles and participation in activities related to them, combined with their greater leisure time unencumbered by responsibility for others, are expressed in the greater prevalence and incidence of road traffic accidents they experience. But also at work in these statistical patterns is men's aggressive differentiation of themselves from women and the affirmation of reproductive difference. As Emslie and Hunt (2008: 808) have commented:

> ... one way in which men can demonstrate culturally valued...forms of 'masculinity' is by denying vulnerability, taking risks which may injure their health and rejecting health beliefs and behaviours which they associate with women.

Yet, it is the combination of gender dynamics with those of class, indigeneity and ethnicity that provides a more complete foundation for understanding the injury and carnage men experience through their involvement with motor vehicles and violence. Criminologists have demonstrated that class is strongly implicated in relation to violence, suicide and homicide (White 2008, Anthony and Cuneen 2008). Precisely how and why is a complex issue, but certainly constraints on access to material, symbolic and agentic resources associated with working-class lives are significant. Limited education is especially significant but undiagnosed and untreated mental impairment and 'disorders', low income, precarious employment or unemployment, substance abuse, family violence and neglect have all been identified as influential (Anthony and Cuneen 2008). Class is also related to road traffic accidents insofar as some of the class factors responsible for working-class men's higher rates of homicide and suicide, especially limited education, are also implicated in their higher rates of injury from motor vehicle accidents (WHO 2010a, Courtney 2011). Yet, the operation of class here also involves the making of masculinity through leisure and recreational activity and the gendered social relations that characterise it. For many working-class men, especially those under 25 years of age with the highest rates of injury and fatality from road traffic accidents, driving motor vehicles is not simply a form of transportation or a means to travel from one place to another. It is a symbolic practice – obviously using material items – through which they establish themselves as part of a *culture* of young working-class men and, in turn, a masculinity that is validated within and by it (Willis 1990, Walker, Butland and Connell 2000). As the injury and death rates associated with the culture show, differentiation from femininity through reckless and high-speed driving, often in displays of competitive masculinity, is intrinsic to this commonly injurious process. Significantly, this class-based pattern of injury among young men is a world-wide phenomenon as the WHO's (2013f) global report on road traffic injuries reported:

> More than 90% of deaths that result from road traffic injuries occur in low- and middle-income countries. Road traffic injury death rates are highest in the low- and middle-income countries of the African and Eastern Mediterranean regions. Even within high-income countries, people from lower socioeconomic backgrounds are more likely to be involved in a road traffic crashes than their more affluent counterparts.

As statistics on the higher rates of incarceration of African-American men in the United States (US Federal Bureau of Prisons 2009) and Indigenous men in Australia (see Chapter 6) also indicate, men from some ethnic minorities share many of the features operating in the lives of working-class men. These see them over-represented in injurious road traffic accidents and violence, especially involving murder, attempted murder and armed robbery. Ethnicity and indigeneity, then, make further additions to the mix of dynamics that produces the adverse health outcomes men from working-class backgrounds experience through their high-risk activities. Racial discrimination (see Chapter 5) and the social dynamics of indigeneity (see Chapter 6), combined with those of class, appear to be the main culprits but much is still to be learnt about how these processes work in generating the rates of injury they inflict.

One of the fields of high-risk practice in which the combination of dynamics of gender and other social division exerts pervasively adverse health impacts is the use of tobacco and illicit drugs, and excessive alcohol consumption. Again, class, marginalised ethnicity or indigeneity combine with masculinity to produce more frequent rates of substance use than other configurations of social dynamics, producing all the attendant diseases and injuries for which such use is well known (WHO 2005a, 2010c, Lang, Greig and Connell 2008, Courtney 2011, Gil and Vega 2010). Working-class African-American and Native American men in the United States, for instance, have the highest substance use rates in that country.

It is of course true that the gap between men's and women's consumption of tobacco and alcohol is closing (Annandale 2003), but class exerts a major force in this convergence as Lorraine Greaves (2007: 116) pointed out in relation to tobacco consumption:

> The remaining smokers in the developed countries are often socially marginalised, of low socioeconomic status and often have other co-occurrent issues such as mental illness and homelessness.

It is among working-class women in high-income countries (Graham et al. 2006) and women in low and middle-income countries (Greaves 2007) that the increased use of tobacco among women is mainly occurring. Meanwhile, the decline in smoking is being led by men from privileged class backgrounds in high-income countries. At the same time, where there is growing evidence of a greater convergence in men's and women's excessive alcohol use, as in Australia, class is also implicated. In this case, the convergence is among younger, middle-class men and women employed in professional occupations (Lindsay 2006). Here, the growing gender equality in some areas of professional employment, such as law and business, is played out after work in licensed premises. New gendered alcohol practices now challenge what was the exclusive preserve of professional men and an arena for work-related masculine differentiation (Wacjman 1999).

Gender inequality and health: Global domestic violence, and childbirth in the Global South

Although, like the pattern for men, there are health differences among women as a result of the combination of gender and other social dynamics such as class, ethnicity and indigeneity, these are generally not as statistically large as those that represent *major health disparities among men,* as documented and discussed above. For example, all-cause mortality rates among Australians aged 25–54 years by sex and occupation in the period 1998–2000 reveal that deaths per 100 000 men in blue-collar occupations or manual jobs amounted to 234, compared with 115 for men in white-collar or middle-class employment (Draper, Turrell and Oldenburg 2004). The rate per 100 000 for blue-collar women was 90, and 80 for their white-collar counterparts. Clearly, class dynamics mean that some groups of women face more adverse health conditions than others, but these health disparities among women, and others related to indigeneity and ethnicity, for example, are generally less pronounced than those experienced among men – at least in the world's high-income countries (WHO 2009b).

Of far greater significance in terms of gender and health disparity are the global gendered dynamics that affect only (or overwhelmingly) women and girls, causing major and even catastrophic health damage to them in the process. These dynamics work across class, ethnicity and indigeneity. To the extent that the damage results predominantly from patriarchal dominance, the health outcomes involved are not simply gendered but an intrinsic feature of gender inequality. Here, the health outcomes arising from men's violence towards women and children are critically important. But the astonishingly high rate of maternal mortality and disability associated with the absence of adequate primary health care for women during pregnancy and childbirth, primarily in sub-Saharan Africa and South Asia, also expresses the operation of patriarchal gender dynamics, particularly in relation to global division (see Chapter 3) and its effects on global health care (see Chapter 8).

In wealthy OECD countries such as Australia, domestic/family violence, or intimate partner violence (IPV), imposes an enormous health toll on women. According to the Australian Human Rights Commission (2012: 7), 'domestic and family violence is the leading contributor to death, disability and illness in women aged 15 to 44 years. It is responsible for more of the disease burden for all women than ... smoking and obesity.' Worldwide, men's violence has affected at least one out of every three women from beatings, sexual coercion and physical abuse (Abdool, Garcia-Moreno and Amin 2012). In 'some countries half to two-thirds of female deaths from violence are by a partner, whereas intimate partners account for only four percent of male homicides' (Abdool et al. 2012: 39). While physical injury is a common outcome of violence for men, a variety of physical, sexual, reproductive and mental health problems are the more likely outcomes for women subjected to men's violence. This is especially marked in South Africa where, based on international incidence rates, rape is perpetrated more commonly than anywhere else in the world (Gilbert and Selikow 2012: 216):

> In 2006, a study reported that close to one in four men surveyed [in South Africa] had participated in sexual violence. Of the total, 16.3 per cent had raped a non-partner or had participated in gang rape, while 8.4 per cent had been sexually violent towards an intimate partner.

In addition, women with violent or controlling male partners, who generally have higher rates of HIV, are more likely to be infected with HIV because their partners tend to impose risky sexual practices (Urdang 2006 cited in Gilbert and Selikow 2012: 216).

There is wide variation in rates of men's violence towards women on a global basis, as the WHO's landmark study (WHO 2005b) of IPV against women and its health effects shows. Conducted in 10 countries, mainly low and middle-income, it found the lowest rates of physical and sexual violence towards women in the high-income country of Japan:

> The proportion of ever-partnered women who had ever experienced physical or sexual violence, or both, by an intimate partner in their lifetime, ranged from 15% [in Japan] to 71%, with most sites falling between 29% and 62%... [T]he greatest amount of violence was reported by women living in ... [mostly rural] settings in Bangladesh, Ethiopia, Peru, and the United Republic of Tanzania. (WHO 2005b: 5)

Most of those who reported such violence usually experienced violent acts more than once and sometimes frequently. The health effects of such experiences consisted mainly of minor physical injuries (bruises, cuts, bites and so on), but in a significant minority of cases, broken bones and eye and ear injuries were also reported (WHO 2005b). In most settings, apart from Japan, Samoa and Tanzania, women who had ever experienced sexual or physical IPV were much more likely to report poor health or very poor health than women who had never experienced such violence. In all settings, sexually or physically abused women were much more likely to have considered or attempted suicide. In most settings, they were also more likely, if they had ever been pregnant, to have suffered higher rates of miscarriages and abortions (WHO 2005b).

The WHO's (2005b) multi-country study of men's violence towards women found that what protected women from such violence in terms of the particular social settings of the participants were: greater economic equality between men and women, women's higher levels of mobility and autonomy, social attitudes expressing opposition to violence against women, intervention by extended family, neighbours and friends in domestic violence incidents, and lower levels of male-on-male aggression and crime. Such settings, however, were not widespread and mainly confined to Japan. It appears, in fact, that a specific combination of gender relations and practices – or gender regime – was largely responsible for the more restricted domestic violence (including IPV) that prevailed in Japan. These relations and practices encompassed greater material equality between women and men, practical social support for non-violent and cooperative relationships between men and women (and among men), and affirmation of women's advancement.

Some have suggested that gendered violence is not simply an expression of patriarchal gender inequality (see Schofield 2012a). They propose that women also engage in IPV against their male partners, inflicting serious injuries.

The evidence used in support of this claim is drawn mainly from large quantitative studies and surveys, predominantly in the United States. The findings of these studies disclose that while men typically express their physical violence towards their intimate partners by strangling them or beating them up, women do so mainly by slapping, punching, kicking, scratching or throwing things. There are, however, some significant limitations in these studies as reputable, research-based critics have noted (Dobash and Dobash 2004). For example, there is an alleged symmetry in men's and women's IPV that derives from a view of violence as discrete 'acts' regardless of who performs them, the circumstances in which they occur and how participants understand what they mean to them. As critics have commented, however:

> [The] 'act-based' approach must invariably equate the physical impact/ consequences of a 'slap' delivered by a slight 5 ft 4 inch woman with the 'slap' of a heavily built man of 6 ft 2 inches. (Dobash and Dobash 2004: 329)

Domestic violence, including IPV, is not the only expression of patriarchal gender dynamics involved in causing major health damage to women and girls, both within and between countries, and on a large scale. In sub-Saharan Africa and South Asia, in particular, the absence of adequate *primary health care* (see Chapter 8) causes astoundingly high maternal mortality rates. For 2013, the world's highest maternal mortality rates – or deaths of women in pregnancy and childbirth for every 100 000 live births – were 510 in sub-Saharan Africa and 190 in South Asia (UNICEF 2014). These compared with a rate of 15 among 'industrialised' or high-income countries. The overall maternal mortality rate for sub-Saharan Africa, of course, masks country-based rates in the region that, while revealing a decline on previous years (WHO 2014a), remain shocking. In Sierra Leone, for instance, the 2013 rate was 1100; in Somalia 850, in South Sudan and the Congo 730 and in Guinea 650. Certainly, hunger and poor nutrition among girls and women, often intensified by regional armed conflict (as in Somalia and South Sudan), have a great effect on maternal mortality in the Global South. Inadequate food and nutrition impede the development and capacity of bodies that can give birth without having to endure major complications and a greater risk of death. Such a situation, however, makes access to primary health care all the more important (see Chapter 8).

In relation to pregnancy and childbirth, primary health care involves regular and close contact between patient and a trained carer, usually in or near the patient's home or workplace. Carers are knowledgeable about and skilled in dealing with pregnancy and childbirth, and establish a relationship with the woman early in her pregnancy. They monitor the pregnancy, providing advice and support, and use only basic medical equipment and birthing technologies to prevent complications and minimise the deaths of mothers and babies. Such care does not demand high-tech hospitals nor specialist medical practitioners. Basically, it requires trained and skilled health care workers who live and work in communities, with back-up by generalist medical practitioners. The lack of such provision, as explained in more detail in Chapter 8, is directly related to the dominance of *market-based,* high-tech medicine that favours cures and complex interventions. It is an approach to health care advanced by male-dominated specialist medicine, global corporations and international financial institutions, and operates mainly out of the Global North and for the 'benefit' of its citizens. This model of health care uses almost all of the world's health care resources, including health care workers, many of whom are 'poached' from the very same regions with the world's highest maternal mortality (see Chapter 8).

There is no question that the problem of maternal mortality in the Global South is related to gender inequality within the countries it encompasses and *their* governments (see Chapter 7). Patriarchal gender dynamics in sub-Saharan Africa and South Asia are responsible for some of the world's most spectacular inequalities – and injustices – between men and women, as we have seen. Yet, just as the inadequate supply of food for the peoples of the Global South is directly linked to global division and class dynamics (see Chapter 3), so, too, is the shortage of primary health care attributable to global division, health care and patriarchal gender dynamics. As discussed further in Chapter 8, male-dominated governments and international financial institutions, such as the World Bank and the International Monetary Fund (IMF), both situated in the global metropole, impose considerable pressure on the governments of the Global South to cut back public provision of health care, including primary care. While explicitly not intended to 'disadvantage women', the health burden of this approach falls disproportionately, and indeed traumatically, on pregnant women in sub-Saharan Africa and South Asia. To the extent that such global social dynamics associated with governance (Chapter 7) and the distribution of health care (Chapter 8) impose most of the health toll they generate on pregnant women of the global periphery, they are inextricably expressions of patriarchal gender inequality.

Conclusions

Gender is a social process that centres on the sexual reproductive distinction. Such differentiation in itself does not necessarily cause social inequality.

Rather, the connection between sex difference and social inequality results from gender dynamics that make the sexual reproductive distinction matter in terms of people's access to material, symbolic and agentic resources.

Gender brings people into being as boys and girls, women and men, and is a key determinant of who gets to do what, when, how, why, with whom and with what consequences in everyday life. In the process, it confers greater benefits on men, both within and between countries, so it inextricably involves the exercise of power. Not that gender operates like a conveyor belt that churns out two variations of its basic model. Nor does it work in such a way that it systematically advantages *all* men at the expense of *all* women, *all* of the time. Rather, it interacts with other processes of social division, generating gendered mixtures of advantage and disadvantage. Nevertheless, it is common for an aggregate or broad pattern of social inequality to be produced by gender dynamics across a range of sites or settings, from organisations and institutions such as the family, corporations and public sector agencies, to whole societies and, indeed, across the globe. The process by which they do so involves a combination of structures of gendered practices.

The dominant approach to gender and health throughout the world is one that focuses on sex differences (male/female) and measurable health outcomes. In aggregate, the picture portrayed by the statistical patterns used in the process suggests that women live longer, sicker lives than men. Men, on the other hand, live shorter lives characterised by more injury and substance use problems, mainly related to consumption of tobacco and alcohol, but also illicit drugs. However, such an approach is based on an understanding of gender as two distinct, biologically based categories of human being – male and female – who basically inhabit mutually exclusive social universes. There is negligible evidence to support this perspective. In fact, while a range of reputable research sources suggests there are some significant differences between the sexes, men and women share many more similarities.

Nevertheless, the prevailing gender order, or the dominant pattern of gender relations throughout the world, both within and between countries, is one of gender inequality and male dominance – or patriarchy. These involve processes of gender division that are characterised by control and exploitation of women, and that return a significantly greater dividend to men as a group. They are evident in many areas of life, including business, politics and government, employment, income and households, in which women do most of the work and care for household members. By contrast with the sex-differences approach to understanding how gender works in relation to health, a gender dynamics approach discloses how the health of men and women involves the exercise of gendered power and inequality and its intersection with other forms of social division. The diverse forms through which this is played out produce multiple and varying gender regimes and patterns of health among and between men and women.

Gendered health means that some groups of men have worse health than others, and the same among women, but that the disparities among men are greater than those among women. However, it does not mean that there is an aggregate pattern of health for men on one side and another for women on the other. Gender inequality and patriarchy nevertheless do produce health disparities between men and women, both within and between countries. One of the most significant involves IPV, whereby men assert power over women at major health expense to women in order to establish masculine superiority and privilege. The other relates mainly to the grave health costs that pregnant women in the Global South incur as a result of male-dominated, market-based health care and financial institutions in the global metropole.

Questions for discussion

1   What distinguishes gender from other processes of social division?
2   Do gender dynamics always involve social inequality?
3   What does it mean to say that gender dynamics are historically and socially variable?
4   How does a sex-differences approach to health characterise the health of men and women?
5   What are the limitations of this approach?
6   What is a gender order and what does it mean to say that it is patriarchal?
7   How robust is the evidence for the claim that gender inequality prevails on a global basis?
8   What is gendered health? What are examples of gender dynamics involved in it?
9   What is the relationship between gender dynamics, intersectionality and health disparity?
10   How are gender inequality and patriarchy evident in health disparity between men and women?

5 Ethnicity and health

Overview   *Christina Ho and Toni Schofield*

- What does the evidence tell us about ethnic disparities in health on a global basis?

- What is 'race'? What does a racist explanation of, or approach to, ethnic disparities in health involve?

- What does it mean to say that ethnicity and ethnic division are social processes? What role does institutional racism play in these?

- How does ethnicity work in the production of ethnic disparities in health?

New York City, approximately 1890

The homes of the Hebrew quarter are its workshops also...You are made fully aware of it before you have travelled the length of a single block in any of these East Side streets, by the whir of a thousand sewing-machines, worked at high pressure from earliest dawn till mind and muscle give out together. Every member of the family, from the youngest to the oldest, bears a hand, shut in the qualmy rooms, where meals are cooked and clothing washed and dried besides, the livelong day. It is not unusual to find a dozen persons – men, women, and children – at work in a single small room...Typhus fever and smallpox are bred here...Filthy diseases both, they sprout naturally among the hordes that bring the germs with them from across the sea... The health officers are on constant and sharp lookout for hidden fever-nests. Considering that half of the ready-made clothes that are sold in the big stores, if not a good deal more than half, are made in these tenement rooms, this is not excessive caution. It has happened more than once that a child recovering from small-pox, and in the most contagious stage of the disease, has been found crawling among heaps of half-finished clothing that the next day would be offered for sale on the counter of a Broadway store; or that a typhus fever patient has been discovered in a room whence perhaps a hundred coats had been sent home that week, each one with the wearer's death-warrant, unseen and unsuspected, basted in the lining (Riis 1890).

The above is a description of the Jewish quarter of New York City in the late 19th century. It was written by journalist and photographer Jacob Riis, in his pioneering book, *How the Other Half Lives* (1890). One of the first to use flash photography, Riis walked through the slums of the Lower East Side, knocking on doors and photographing inhabitants and their squalid living conditions. Jews and other immigrants lived in hopelessly overcrowded tenements without heating, running water or garbage disposal, and epidemics of cholera and other infectious diseases were often traced back to their neighbourhoods. Riis spent years documenting New York City's slum life, assuming that if only wealthier New Yorkers realised how their fellow city-dwellers lived, they would be moved to action.

However, at this time, debates raged between social reformers like Riis, who argued that disease-infested immigrant neighbourhoods needed practical refurbishments like air shafts and sewers, and those who insisted that filth and disease were part of the immigrants' moral degeneracy. Another reformer, anthropologist Franz Boas (1912), found that a new environment, and new jobs and diets, actually altered the physical bodies of immigrants. Differences between immigrants and citizens were therefore environmental, not biological, he argued. This history of New York City's slums is a powerful reminder of how health and disease are intimately linked to broader social processes and the divisions and conflicts that characterise them.

While previous chapters have explained how class and gender combine to produce health inequities, this chapter turns to the story of ethnicity and health. It shows how class and gender interact with ethnicity to produce complex social outcomes. As the history of New York City shows, the health of ethnic minorities is often dramatically different to that of majority populations. And still today, all around the world, with a few notable exceptions (see below), disparities in health are a major feature of the differences between ethnic groups, with ethnic minorities having poorer health than majority populations. This is evident in all manner of health indicators, with often large differences in life expectancy, infant mortality, rates of cancers and heart disease, just to name a few.

This chapter explains that ethnic disparities in health, like disparities explored in previous chapters, are predominantly the products of social processes that produce inequality. While those associated with ethnicity mix and merge with class and gender, they are nevertheless distinct from them. They are a specific social domain related to a combination of social practices and heritage that distinguish groups of people as 'culturally' distinct from each other, such as their history, religion, language, physical appearance, styles of dress, food and music, and ceremonial occasions associated with major life events such as birth, marriage and death. Ethnic division arises when the practices and features of an ethnic group are made to matter in ways that impose major and enduring barriers to material, symbolic and agentic resources (see Chapter 3). It is through this process that ethnic minorities are brought into being. We will return to this point below. But first, let's take a look at the scope of ethnic disparities in health.

Documenting ethnic disparities in health

While the history of New York City shows the appalling living conditions endured by immigrants in the 19th century, ethnic inequalities continue to plague American society today. For example, Black men in poor areas have 20 years' shorter life expectancy than richer White men (Marmot 2006). Meanwhile, African-Americans and Hispanics have higher rates of heart disease, strokes, diabetes, HIV/AIDS and infant mortality, when compared to the White population (Bhopal 2007). Basic health indicators in various high-income countries show that these inequalities are not confined to the United States. In the United Kingdom, most ethnic groups originating beyond its shores have higher mortality rates than the general population, and increased rates of diseases like tuberculosis, malaria, diabetes and hypertension (Drever and Whitehead 1997; Bhopal 2007). In the Netherlands, the mortality rate of Turkish and Moroccan immigrant children under 15 years is two to three times higher than that for Dutch-born children (Schulpen 1996).

Even in low to middle-income countries, a similar pattern of health by ethnicity is evident. In China, infant mortality rates among some ethnic minorities are more than twice the national average (Kabeer 2006). In India, the infant mortality rate among *dalit*, or 'untouchable', castes is 83 per 1000 live births, compared to only 68 for other groups (Kabeer 2006). In Vietnam, ethnic minority women face a four times higher risk of maternal mortality compared to majority Kinh women (Malqvist et al. 2013). Across Asia, similar ethnic disparities can be seen for indicators such as underweight children, malnutrition and maternal mortality (Kabeer 2006).

It should be noted, however, that in some cases, ethnic minorities have better health than majority populations. The 'healthy migrant effect' describes the superior health of migrants upon arrival. For example, overseas-born people in Australia generally experience mortality rates 10 to 15 per cent lower than for Australian-born persons, and have lower rates of hospitalisation, disability and 'lifestyle'-related risk factors, such as heavy alcohol use and smoking

(Singh and de Looper 2002: 1). In part this is due to healthy individuals self-selecting for migration, and also because of the health requirements of the country's migration program. Asian-born immigrants have death rates up to 40 per cent lower than the native-born, with those born in Vietnam, the Philippines, China and Malaysia exhibiting the lowest rates (AIHW 2010).

Similarly, in the United Kingdom, there are some conditions that are less common among minority groups, including many cancers (particularly lung and breast cancers), anxiety and depressive disorders, suicide, peripheral vascular disease and alcoholism (Bhopal 2007). In the United States, ethnic minorities have also been found to exhibit better mental health than the majority population, partly due to the protective effects of religious participation and strong family bonds (Nazroo and Williams 2006: 258).

However, the 'healthy migrant effect' wanes over time, and immigrants can experience a quicker deterioration in health than native-born residents. In Australia, research has shown that after about 20 years, there is generally no health gap between immigrants and the native born (Kennedy and McDonald 2006). A similar pattern prevails in Canada (Gushulak et al. 2011). It is not clear why this occurs. To date no comprehensive longitudinal research has examined the relationship between length of residence after migration, access to social resources and health patterns. However, in Australia, there is strong evidence indicating a correlation between the location over time of non-English speaking immigrants in the most health-damaging and precarious employment, combined with other class and gender-related constraints (see Chapters 3 and 4), and deteriorating health (Schofield 1990, Alcorso and Schofield 1991). Recent evidence on labour force participation suggests markedly higher rates of both unemployment and participation in low-paid, health-damaging jobs among recently arrived immigrants, compared to the Australian-born and those from the 'main English-speaking countries' (Birrell and Healy 2013). We will return to this later in the chapter.

Health patterns, then, obviously vary between ethnic groups. And even within ethnic minorities there may be different patterns of disease and disability. For example, South Asians in the United Kingdom generally have a low prevalence of smoking, but Bangladeshi men have an extremely high one (Bhopal 2007). Nevertheless, on the whole, ethnic minorities fare worse than majority populations on many important health indicators.

In addition, where universal health insurance does not prevail (see Chapter 8), ethnic minorities typically face significantly greater barriers to accessing health care and health insurance. In many countries around the world, ethnic minorities make less use of health services than majority groups. In the United States, where most research on this issue has been conducted to date, study after study has shown that ethnic minorities are less likely than White Americans to have health insurance, and have greater difficulty getting health care, and have fewer choices in where to receive care (Smedley, Stith and Nelson 2003). This often translates into some startling statistics. For example, African-Americans have 50 per cent higher odds of an in-hospital death, compared to White Americans (Chandra 2009). In 1999, an extensive study commissioned by the American Congress concluded that ethnic disparities are 'consistent and extensive across a range of medical conditions and healthcare services, are associated with worse health outcomes, and occur independently of insurance status, income, and education, among other factors that influence access to healthcare' (Smedley, Stith and Nelson 2003: 79).

In most high-income countries, health care systems do not cater for all ethnic groups in an equivalent manner. Even when minority groups do seek to access medical help, as British sociologist Anthony Giddens (2009) noted, language barriers can prevent adequate communication, and culturally specific understandings of health, illness, treatment and death are often not considered by health professionals. In-patient facilities may not offer appropriate food for people of all cultural backgrounds or facilities to pray or perform appropriate ablutions. Not having access to a health professional of the same gender may prohibit some individuals from ethnic minorities from accessing care (Bhopal 2007). Such inadequacies reflect the fact that health services are largely planned and managed by members of majority populations, based on an implicit understanding of the needs and preferences of patients (Bhopal 2007). Evidence from the United Kingdom shows that in primary care, members of ethnic minorities are more likely to be dissatisfied about aspects of the care received, to wait longer for an appointment and to face language barriers during the consultation (Nazroo 2014).

Consequently, members of ethnic minorities generally participate less in health services when compared with the majority population. For example, Australian research in 2007 showed that people who mainly spoke a language other than English were less likely than English speakers to have used health services in the previous 12 months for a lifetime mental disorder (26 per 100 000 population compared with 48). Meanwhile, in 2005–06, women in the target breast-screening population (50–69 years) who spoke a non-English language were less likely than their English-speaking counterparts to participate in breast screening (45 per cent and 59 per cent, respectively; AIHW 2010).

Moving beyond the Global North, we find that ethnic disparities in access to health care are even worse. In many countries in the Global South, ethnic minorities are concentrated in rural and remote areas, with less access to basic health care. Not only are there fewer health facilities within a reasonable distance, but health professionals are often reluctant to work in rural areas, leaving posts vacant for long periods, sometimes resulting in the closure of services. In sub-Saharan Africa, 'many remote regions and districts do not have a single doctor, nurse or midwife to provide assistance to those that need it most' (World Bank 2008). For example, in Malawi, 87 per cent of the population live in rural areas, but 97 per cent of doctors are found in urban health facilities (World Bank 2008). As a consequence, despite all governments' formal commitment to universal primary health care across sub-Saharan Africa, there are striking disparities in the use of health services between ethnic groups (Brockerhoff and Hewett 2000). Citing an all-too-common scenario in the Global South, a journalist in an Indian magazine discussed the situation in one of India's rural areas:

> Ironically, cellphone reaches the tribals in Tamil Nadu's hills, but not healthcare. At 1,800 metres in Siraikkadu forest of Western Ghats, mobile phones ring loud in the serene atmosphere but lack of access to healthcare facilities are taking a toll on the health of the inhabitants there. (Kumar 2013)

As the journalist also explained, most of the women and children in the tribal hill areas suffered from anaemia. And because of a lack of transportation, residents needed to walk at least eight kilometres to the nearest hospital. Even there, doctors were not always available (Kumar 2013).

As Williams and Mohammed (2013: 1214) have noted, access to primary care is associated with smaller social disparities in health, and probably explains the 'unexpectedly good health profiles' of Cuba and Costa Rica (see Chapter 8). The introduction of a community based primary care system in Iran has also reduced health disparities. In two decades Iran has erased a two-fold elevated risk of infant mortality in rural areas compared to urban areas (Williams and Mohammed 2013). These kinds of developments are discussed more fully in Chapter 8.

Why do such ethnic disparities in health exist all over the world? The rest of this chapter explores the ways in which ethnicity is a social process – especially that associated with the production of ethnic division – that is the major driver in this global phenomenon.

'Race', biology and health

As previous chapters have explained, and as we saw at the beginning of this chapter in the debates about immigrants in 19th-century New York City, there is a long tradition of viewing health problems as reflecting biological susceptibility to disease and illness. Immigrants in the United States were historically considered to be inherently degenerate, resulting in their high rates of disease and death. Meanwhile, 'negroes' were thought to be biologically susceptible to diseases like leprosy, tetanus, pneumonia, scurvy and sore eyes (Bhopal 2007).

Many of these ideas have since been discredited, though genetic factors do play a modest role in shaping health outcomes. For example, there is evidence that certain genetic disorders, such as cystic fibrosis and sickle-cell anaemia, may be more prevalent among some ethnic groups than others (Bloom 1995). In recent years, with the advances of the human genome project, biological explanations for ethnic disparities in health have again become more prominent. Scientists have sought to uncover genetic causes of diseases, and we now hear media reports about the 'cancer gene', the 'stress gene' and the 'arthritis gene', among others.

However, genetic differences do not adequately explain ethnic disparities in health. For example, in the United States, the prevalence of hypertension and diabetes is two to three times higher among African-Americans than among the White population. However, in West Africa and among African-origin populations in the Caribbean, rates of these diseases are two to five times lower than those of Black Americans or Black Britons (Kawachi, Daniels and Robinson 2005). Similarly, South Asians in numerous countries have higher rates of heart disease than those on the Indian sub-continent. While heart disease has been comparatively rare in South Asia, in the United Kingdom South Asian immigrants have mortality rates from heart disease 40 to 50 per cent higher than those of the overall population (Bhopal 2007).

Genes obviously do not provide an adequate explanation for ethnic disparities in health. The difficulty with biological approaches is their assumption that different groups of people can be defined by their biological 'race'. Indeed, the concept of 'race' itself is a major barrier to understanding ethnic differences. Even though 'race' is a key concept in the imagination of contemporary societies, it has no clearly agreed-upon definition. 'Race' can refer to birthplace, ancestry, nationality, language or religion, as the following suggests.

Census-taking and changing categories of 'race'

In the United States, the categories used in the Census to count population groups by 'race' have changed at almost every Census since the first one in 1790 (Nazroo and Williams 2006). In the Australian Census, at least four different questions are used, including country of birth, mother's and father's country of birth, language spoken at home and ancestry. While many countries' census questions on ethnicity might include 'Chinese' as an option, in Singapore, the 'Chinese' category lists 22 sub-categories, including Hokkien, Teochew, Cantonese, Hakka, Hainanese and so on. Meanwhile, the 'Indian' category lists 24 sub-categories, including Tamil, Malayali, Punjabi, Bengali and so on (Bhopal 2007). These differences in how national governments classify their populations point to the socially constructed nature of 'race'.

In fact, there is no such thing as 'race' or 'races', in the sense that there is no group of people who can be identified as being any more or less evolved than any other (Russell and Schofield 1986). There is only one 'human race' – *homo sapiens*. But what about the obvious observable physical differences between 'Asiatic', 'Caucasian' and 'Negroid' peoples? Certainly, there are physical differences by blood groups and genetics – accounting for phenotypical traits such as skin or hair colour, shape of eyes or nose, and so on. Yet, 'well over 90 per cent of genetic endowment is similar for all humans' (Trowler 1984: 63). The biological differences that do exist between peoples create no significant variations in terms of human thought and behaviour. Many other differences are considered to be ecological; a result of the evolution of humans adapting to their environment. For example, dark skin provides selective advantage in tropical regions (Blakey 1999), but such theorisation remains speculative.

'Race' and the alleged biological inequalities accompanying it have legitimated colonialism, slavery and other non-democratic systems of governance (see Chapter 6). At the heart of its meaning was that only a minority of the Earth's peoples was biologically suited to governing their own lives. The rest needed to be ruled over. 'Race science' was an attempt to justify these beliefs on 'rational' grounds, culminating in Nazi Germany and the Holocaust in World War II. Meanwhile, in Asia, elements of Western 'race science' were taken up in Japan, China, India and Malaysia (Smedley and Smedley 2005). Even in Central and South America, where there had been extensive mixtures of peoples over centuries of colonisation, in the late 19th and 20th centuries, light skin gradually came to be privileged (Smedley and Smedley 2005).

Following the horror of the Holocaust, 'race science' was discredited, and scientists argued that 'race' had no basis in biology. In the 1950s and 60s, UNESCO released a series of statements showing that racial biology had nothing to do with variation in human thought and behaviour, and that the concept of 'race' was questionable. A statement from the 1950 Paris meeting argued that 'race' is much less a biological phenomenon than an enduring social myth (Montagu 1972). Accordingly, in the social sciences 'race' is often written in quotation marks to remind us that it is a social construction, not a biological reality.

Even if 'race' is a scientifically discredited concept, in practice, people still act as though it is a biological reality. This partly explains why racism continues to exist. For example, 'racial profiling' is often used by police to identify individuals. In Australia, for example, this recently sparked a debate over the term 'of Middle-Eastern appearance', which is regularly used by police and in the media. As Joseph Wakim (2006: 15), founder of the Australian Arabic Council, wrote:

> How can people from more than twenty different countries, from West Africa to West Asia, from Morocco to Medina, share a homogenous physical appearance? Can police seriously be expected to discern between a Syrian, a Cypriot, a Maltese and a Brazilian?

In this example, racial profiling of people 'of Middle Eastern' appearance aligns with widespread suspicion and fear of Arabs and Muslims in many high-income countries in the post-9/11 era, after the terrorist attacks on the United States in 2001. Symbols of cultural difference, such as a Muslim woman's veil or a Muslim man's beard, have taken on a new significance, bringing a heightened visibility to and mistrust of members of ethnic minorities who can be 'identified' as Arab or Muslim. As the next section explains, social divisions arise when aspects of cultural difference are made to matter, and people are treated unequally as a result.

Ethnicity and the social creation of disparities in health

With the discrediting of 'race', social scientists have opted increasingly for the concept of ethnicity to explain cultural difference and inequality. A popular British sociological definition proposes that ethnicity refers to 'the cultural practices and outlooks of a given community of people which sets them apart from others' (Giddens 2009: 633). Further, it proposes that the differences be-tween people are not innate but, rather, produced through social action and in-teraction whereby people 'assimilate the lifestyles, norms and beliefs of ethnic communities' (Giddens 2009: 633).

The social construction of ethnic identity

Even people's understandings of their own ethnic and cultural identities are subject to change. For example, in recent decades, and especially after 9/11 and the War on Terror, there has been much evidence of an 'Islamic re-assertion' among some immigrants in Western societies (Dwyer 2000, Husain and O'Brien 2000, Modood 1990). Growing numbers of Muslim women have taken up the headscarf and other forms of veiling, and attendance at mosques and Islamic schools is rising (for example, Grossman 2012, McNeilage 2013). This prioritising of an Islamic identity (sometimes over and above an ethnic or national identity) can be seen as a response to the discrimination experienced by Muslims in recent decades, an expression of pride and resistance in a hostile environment.

However, not all Muslims deliberately choose to emphasise their religious identity. For example, in discussing her childhood in Australia on national radio, Alyena Mohummadally explained that after 9/11 a Muslim identity was imposed upon her, whereas prior to that she had never been made to feel inferior or threatening:

> When I grew up in the 80s and 90s, being Muslim was only a point of difference amongst my friends, it wasn't a point of fear. There was nothing like the world is nowadays... I was surrounded by people who didn't really care so much, were more like, oh you don't eat pork, oh, you don't drink. But then I'd be like, oh, you give up things for Lent, oh, why do you eat fish on Fridays? So it was a world in which I never really felt Muslim... I felt Pakistani only in so far as every year I visited my grandparents. But for all intents and purposes, I was an Aussie kid... Our brown skin did not distinguish us. (transcribed from Mohummadally 2014)

The fluidity and dynamism of ethnicity explain how ethnic divisions arise, as societies come to classify certain cultural traits and practices as threatening or subordinate. This is how ethnic hierarchies are created, reflecting both histori-cal contexts, such as slavery and colonialism, and contemporary circumstances, such as the War on Terror that began after the 9/11 terrorist attacks in 2001. Ethnic disparities in health reflect these hierarchies between majority and mi-nority populations. We should note that ethnic minorities are not always nu-merically smaller, but are socially and politically inferior to the dominant eth-nicity or ethnicities, and have more limited access to the resources needed to participate adequately in social life. Inferior health is an embodied reflection of this inferior access to social resources.

In many countries, ethnic minorities are more likely to live in poverty than the population at large. In the United States, African-Americans have 2.5 times the poverty rate of White Americans (Kawachi, Daniels and Robinson 2005). And, as discussed above, in many countries ethnic minorities are concentrated in poorer, remote regions. For example, one study in Sichuan Province, China, documented that the average income of ethnic minorities was less than one-tenth the national average (Yuan 2012). People living in poverty are more likely to live in substandard or overcrowded housing in poor neighbourhoods. They may have less access to nutritious foods, good-quality recreational facilities and other services that help to maintain a 'healthy lifestyle'. As such, they are less likely to reduce harmful practices, such as smoking and unhealthy diets. And, as discussed above, they are less likely to be covered by health insurance or have access to adequate and appropriate health care.

It is evident, then, that in many and diverse parts of the globe, ethnic minorities experience remarkably similar constraints on access to social resources associated with health. At the heart of this experience is a social process that makes the 'markers' of ethnicity matter in terms of this access. The main component of this process is *institutional racism*. This term refers to discrimination that 'pervades all of society's structures in a systematic manner' (Giddens 2009: 638), favouring some groups while excluding or penalising others on the basis of their ethnicity. Institutional racism operates through the everyday practices of organisations that comprise education, health care and legal systems, and the employment and housing markets. The 'racial profiling' used by police in Australia, as previously mentioned, exemplifies its operation in the Australian legal system. It is arguably even more pronounced in relation to Australia's Indigenous peoples, as the following chapter shows.

Institutional racism explains why in the United States, for example, even within the same occupational group, White Americans have higher incomes than African-Americans. And within income strata, African-Americans have considerably lower levels of wealth, and are less likely to be home owners. Among those living below the poverty line, African-Americans are more likely than White Americans to remain in this situation over their lifetime (Nazroo and Williams 2006). In the United Kingdom, Pakistani and Bangladeshi immigrants in professional or managerial groups earn an average income equivalent to White people in semi-skilled and unskilled manual classes (Nazroo 2014).

Although racism is often recognised at the level of the individual, and acts of discrimination (and fear of discrimination) have been associated with poorer physical and mental health (Nazroo 2014), institutional racism can have far greater consequences because it operates structurally. In other words, its practices establish collectively differentiated patterns of opportunities and barriers related to social resources, according to ethnicity. As a result, some ethnicities are winners and others losers. Like class dynamics, those of ethnic division are relational. Yet, by contrast with class, the marginalisation and exclusion that characterise it operate through the prism of race.

Institutional racism explains in part why the 'healthy migrant effect' dissipates over time, leading to what has been termed the 'exhausted migrant' effect (Agudelo-Suárez, Ronda-Pérez and Benavides 2011: 162). In countries around the world, immigrants face discrimination in numerous areas of social life, producing detrimental effects on health. Even highly educated immigrants can find their qualifications and experience are not recognised in their new communities, or encounter discrimination from employers, leading to downward career progression, under-employment or unemployment (for evidence from Australia, see Ho and Alcorso 2004, Booth, Leigh and Varganova 2012).

In high-income countries, the stereotypes of the Indian engineer driving taxis and the Russian professor cleaning offices are symbolic of the operation of institutional racism. Around the world, migrant workers tend to be found in low-skill, high-risk jobs, even when their qualifications should secure them better jobs (Agudelo-Suárez, Ronda-Pérez and Benavides 2011). This employment profile leads to higher rates of industrial accidents and workplace deaths among migrants, as well as limiting their options in relation to housing, education, and access to health services (see, for example, Lee, McGuinness and Kawakami 2011). Meanwhile, female migrants employed as domestic workers often report high levels of physical, sexual and psychological abuse (International Organization for Migration (IOM) 2013: 40). Workplace discrimination and gender inequalities combine to channel migrants into what has been labelled the '3D jobs' – 'dirty, demanding and dangerous' (Agudelo-Suárez, Ronda-Pérez and Benavides 2011: 157).

Given these experiences, it is no surprise that migrants' health deteriorates over time in the host society. Sometimes for the first time in their lives, migrants find themselves 'racialised' or defined as an ethnic minority. Their language, customs, beliefs and their bodies are suddenly defined as different from the mainstream, and they are treated accordingly. Even those who have been admitted to the country as skilled migrants, selected for their capacity to contribute to the economy and society, can find themselves in the position of a subordinate ethnic 'other'. In this way, practices of discrimination, marginalisation and exclusion bring ethnicity into being and in profoundly embodied ways, as the research on ethnic health disparities shows.

However, institutional racism does not just operate in relation to the process of migration. Ethnic minorities who have been residents and citizens of a specific country for generations can also face racism in entrenched forms. The experience of African-Americans in the United States is an illustrative case in point. Medical research often blames 'unhealthy lifestyles' for African-Americans' poor health when compared to White Americans', but, as we have seen above, African-Americans' access to the material, symbolic and agentic resources associated with good health is markedly more restricted. For example, African-Americans tend to live in poorer neighbourhoods offering less health-conducive amenity because they have significantly lower incomes. However, access to financial resources is by no means the only or main social factor operating here, as the following explains.

Residential segregation in the United States is a major racialising dimension between White Americans and African-Americans. It seeks to ensure that Black and White Americans live in different neighbourhoods, and is a product of historic and contemporary discrimination. While outright segregation is now illegal in the United States, housing patterns continue to display the legacy of previous practices, such as the 'Jim Crow' laws, enacted between 1876 and 1965, which enforced racial segregation in housing, schools, public places and public transport, as well as in restaurants and restrooms (see Woodward 2002). Additionally, the Federal Housing Administration's historic policy of 'redlining', or coding the credit-worthiness of neighbourhoods based partly on race, meant that residents of Black 'redlined' neighbourhoods were unable to obtain mortgages from banks, and these neighbourhoods suffered significant disinvestment from private institutions (Massey and Denton 1993: 51–52).

While there has been a trend toward desegregation since the 1960s, African-Americans remain the most segregated group in the United States, particularly in large cities such as Chicago, Los Angeles and New York, where they are concentrated in inner-city ghettoes (Denton 2006). Housing discrimination continues today through the practices of real estate agents, landlords and lending institutions, who may provide differential treatment to clients on the basis of their ethnicity, including refusing to rent or sell a property to people of certain ethnicities (Williams and Jackson 2005: 331).

In many aspects, residential segregation applies regardless of class. As Williams and Jackson (2005: 328) have noted, 'middle-class blacks live in poorer areas than whites of similar economic status, and poor whites live in much better neighbourhoods than poor blacks'. This means that Black and White communities have very different experiences of the quality of services and facilities in their local area. For instance, neighbourhoods vary in their provision of recreational facilities and open, green spaces, which shapes individuals' habits around physical exercise. In addition, people who perceive their neighbourhoods to be unsafe are less likely to engage in outdoor activity (Williams and Jackson 2005). In poorer neighbourhoods, it is more difficult to find nutritious products in local convenience stores, shops and supermarkets than in more affluent neighbourhoods. Those in minority and poor neighbourhoods are less likely to offer as wide a variety of food choices as those found in higher-income neighbourhoods (Acevedo-Garcia et al. 2008). Environmental health risks, such as degradation, air, water and soil pollution, and other physical health hazards, are also more prevalent in poorer neighbourhoods (Smedley, Stith and Nelson 2003).

Acevedo-Garcia and colleagues' (2008) study of ethnic disparities in child health noted that 'disadvantaged neighbourhoods' are associated with detrimental health outcomes, negative health behaviour, developmental delays, teen parenthood and academic failure (323). Overall, ethnic minorities have less access to 'opportunity neighbourhoods', defined as those that support healthy development. Opportunity neighbourhoods have good schools and after-school programs, safe streets and playgrounds, and 'positive role models' (Acevedo-Garcia et al. 2008: 323). It should be noted, however, that while 'disadvantaged neighbourhoods' may be lacking in 'opportunity', evidence from the United Kingdom shows that ethnic residential concentration can have benefits for mental health. Living in a neighbourhood with others of the same ethnicity can mean increased social support and lower exposure to racial harassment and discrimination, increasing people's sense of security (Nazroo 2014). Nevertheless, in the United States, programs designed to improve neighbourhood and housing quality have been shown to enhance participants' health. Williams and Mohammed (2013) reported on two such interventions, showing that providing public housing residents access to better housing conditions resulted in better health, including less substance abuse, lower rates of obesity and diabetes risk, and higher levels of mental health and subjective well-being.

Conclusions

In the world's richest society – and one of its most ethnically diverse – the division between the dominant ethnic majority and its second-largest ethnic minority (of African-Americans) demonstrates a pervasive global trend: of a significant health disparity between ethnic minorities and their dominant ethnic counterparts. The poorer health of African-Americans, as we have explained throughout this chapter, is largely the result of institutional racism that operates through systematic marginalisation and exclusion from access to the material, symbolic and agentic resources that is required for people's health. Combined with additional evidence from diverse national sources on ethnic health disparities, this chapter concludes that it is this social process that lies at the heart of what we understand by ethnicity in the production of health inequalities.

The poorer health of ethnic minorities, then, is caused not by genetics, nor by 'unhealthy' cultural practices. Rather, it is the outcome of a combination of divisive social processes – including class and gender – but in which ethnicity plays a distinct role in imposing constraints on access to the social resources needed for health. The creation of ethnic divisions operates through social practices that transform the cultural features of a group into formidable barriers to resources and the poor health that accompanies them. Whether African-Americans struggling with their country's highest rates of unemployment, lowest-paid jobs and worst housing and neighbourhood amenity, or new immigrants trapped in hazardous and precarious jobs with more limited access to appropriate health care in high-income countries, or the armies of ethnic minorities concentrated in the poorest regions of rural China or India, they all share a social dynamic that is played out through their bodies. Not all suffer its damaging effects but, as the growing evidence shows, ethnicity is a domain of social process that creates divisions among people based on what are quintessential, taken-for-granted features of who they are, how they live and how they make sense of the world.

Questions for discussion

1 What are some of the main indicators of ethnic differences in health?
2 Why has 'race' been discredited in explaining ethnic differences and disparities in health?

3   What do you understand by the concept of ethnicity from a sociological perspective?
4   How does ethnicity differ from ethnic division?
5   Where do ethnic minorities come from?
6   What is institutional racism? What role does it play in ethnic disparities in health?

6 Indigeneity and health

Overview   *Toni Schofield and John Gilroy*

- What are the main health effects of indigeneity?

- How might 'indigeneity' refer to a social process? How is 'coercive alienation' central to understanding it?

- What is the relationship between colonisation and global division in relation to indigeneity? How does it work?

- How do the health experiences of Indigenous Australians illuminate the dynamics of indigeneity?

Northern Queensland, Australia, 1870s

This morning in the predawn dark, his eyes accustomed to darkness, Bidiggi could see the white men's own totemic circle of saddles and packs stacked to make a *bora* ring. Behind that little wall he knew, and his father and uncles and brothers knew, the white man lay in wait...

[H]e raced forward with his spear...Then the shouting sticks began to bark... His brother crumpled like a broken tree...

[H]e could see as the dark thinned that more and more of his tribe had fallen...He shook with fear...

The remnants of the tribe were in flight...The world was a madness of shouts and the drumming of the animals, the screams of the running men.

Two old men...had been left behind, and their wives. The other women had been shot as they fled. The old women wailed and were silenced...

Bidiggi was only twelve, and although he didn't measure by white time but by black, he knew he was a man. There had been the ceremony. His father was dead. His brother. His uncles...His head filled with pictures of the men on the big animals beating the tribe like wild pigs along the reedy rim of the water where they fished and swam. The pictures were blotted with blood and he could still hear the men screaming back when the shouting sticks spoke to them and see the running women and children trampled into the morning grass. (Astley 1987: 39–41)

As the above extract from Thea Astley's (1987) novel suggests, indigeneity has a bloody history. It is also a history of continuing collective trauma transmitted over many years and across many generations. Indigeneity reverberates in the embodied intergenerational experience of its survivors as shortened life expectancy, chronic illness and disability (Alderete et al. 1999, Pulver et al. 2010, Gilroy et al. 2013). Understanding *how* and *why* these traumatic events occurred requires understanding of how indigeneity works as a social process and as a group identity. Before we do this, however, the following surveys what research and other evidence reveal about a significant dimension of the embodied experience of indigeneity through measurable health outcomes across the globe.

Indigenous peoples' health: Global snapshots

In 1999, the World Health Organization (WHO) reported that there were around 370 million Indigenous peoples living in at least 70 countries across the world. Around 7 million of these resided in high-income countries, such as Australia, Canada, New Zealand, the Scandinavian region and the United States. According to the WHO report:

> Indigenous peoples are over represented among the poor, and their living conditions and health status are invariably below those of the general population of each country. Their health status is severely affected by low income levels, and by low availability of safe water, food, sanitation and access to health services. One of the main threats, not only to their health, but to their very survival, is the destruction of their habitat, which provides spiritual and material sustenance. (Alderete et al. 1999: i)

The following statistical snapshots illustrate the breadth and severity of this situation.

Life-expectancy rates

The WHO (Alderete et al. 1999, Pulver et al. 2010) has identified a 'life-expectancy gap' between Indigenous and non-Indigenous peoples of 5–20 years. However, life expectancy for some Indigenous peoples, such as those in sub-Saharan Africa, is markedly worse than most others throughout the world (Ohenjo et al. 2006, Alderete et al. 1999, Alderete 1999). The life-expectancy gap between Indigenous and non-Indigenous peoples in high-income countries for which there are recent data (2001–13) indicates a range of 3–13 years.

TABLE 6.1 *Life-expectancy rates by age for Indigenous and non-Indigenous peoples in Australia, Canada, New Zealand and United States*

COUNTRY X YEAR(S)	INDIGENOUS PEOPLE	LIFE EXPECTANCY OF INDIGENOUS (YEARS)	LIFE EXPECTANCY OF NON-INDIGENOUS (YEARS)	LIFE-EXPECTANCY GAP (YEARS)
Australia (2008)	Aboriginal and Torres Strait Islanders	71.40	81.40	10.00
Canada (2001 projections to 2017)	a) First Nations	a) 75.85	a) 81.00	a) 5.15
	b) Métis	b) 77.00	b) 81.00	b) 4.00
	c) Inuit	c) 68.50	c) 81.00	c) 12.50
New Zealand (2012)	Māori	74.65	81.95	7.30
United States (2011)	Native Indian	75.10	78.70	3.62

Sources: Compiled from AIHW 2011a, Claude et al. 2005, Statistics New Zealand 2013, Lewis, Burd-Sharps and Sachs 2010.

As Table 6.1 shows, Indigenous peoples have a lower life expectancy than non-Indigenous peoples in the four wealthy nations of Australia, Canada, New Zealand and the United States. The biggest gaps in life expectancy between Indigenous and non-Indigenous peoples occur in Australia and Canada.

Low birth-weight and foetal death rates

Indigenous peoples generally have higher rates of low birth-weight babies and foetal deaths than non-Indigenous peoples. Low birth-weight occurs when a baby is born, at term, weighing less than 2.5 kilograms, which generally indicates conditions of social impoverishment and stress on the mother (see Chapter 3). Table 6.2 shows the number of foetal deaths per 1000 live births and low birth-weight babies per 100 live births among Indigenous and non-Indigenous peoples of the United States, New Zealand and Australia. In both Australia and the United States, Indigenous foetal death rates are worse than their non-Indigenous counterparts. In New Zealand, while there is little difference between foetal mortality rates among Māori and non-Māori groups, Māori experience lower birth-weight than non-Māori. Australian Indigenous peoples' rate of low birth-weight is twice that of non-Indigenous Australians. The rates of foetal death and low birth-weight taken together suggest that Indigenous Australians' birth outcomes are the worst of all Indigenous peoples in the three selected high-income countries. However, comparisons *between* countries and peoples are indicative only. They represent general trends rather than exact rates of difference, because the years for which the data apply vary.

TABLE 6.2 *Foetal deaths per 1000 live births and low birth-weight per 100 live births, various years*

COUNTRY	INDIGENOUS PEOPLE	FOETAL DEATHS		LOW BIRTH-WEIGHT (2.5 KG)	
		INDIGENOUS	NON-INDIGENOUS	INDIGENOUS	NON-INDIGENOUS
United States	Native Indian	8.5[*]	5.3[*^]	7.5[**]	7.1[**]
New Zealand	Māori	8[***]	6.4[***]	7.6[***]	5.5[***]
Australia	Aboriginal & Torres Strait Islanders	11.1[^^]	7.1[^^]	12[^^^]	6[^^^]

Sources: Compiled from US Department of Health and Human Services 2013, New Zealand Ministry of Health 2013, AIHW 2011a, MacDorman, Kirmeyer and Wilson 2012.

[*] 1995–2006
[^] This figure is for non-Hispanic/White population
[**] 2011
[***] 2010
[^^] 2004–08
[^^^] 2007

'Lifestyle factors'

'Lifestyle factors' are epidemiological measures of behaviours and bodily conditions that are strongly associated with chronic diseases, health conditions and infectious diseases, such as heart disease, stroke and diabetes. The term 'lifestyle factors' is problematic because it suggests that population-based patterns of health outcomes are primarily related to 'individual behaviours', rather than to structural social processes, as discussed in previous chapters. Understanding indigeneity as a social process means seeing these 'lifestyle factors' as statistical indicators rather than causes of health-damaging practices. Such factors include, but are not confined to, limited physical activity, sedentary work, cigarette smoking, poor nutrition, alcohol misuse and substance abuse. They are common features of Indigenous life that have embodied effects such as high rates of illness and disease (Stoner, Stoner and Fryer 2012).

Cigarette smoking

Tobacco use is associated with the cultural and ceremonial practices of many Indigenous peoples, such as in the Americas. In some Indigenous communities, engaging in tobacco use is a gateway to adulthood and ceremony (Steele et al. 2008, Alderete et al. 2010). The rate of cigarette smoking on a regular basis among most Indigenous peoples, however, is significantly greater than non-Indigenous peoples in most countries around the world. For example, the rate of tobacco use among the Indigenous peoples of New Zealand and Australia is around double that of their non-Indigenous counterparts in those countries (Cook 2013, AIHW 2011b).

Alcohol consumption

Alcohol consumption is not only a leading cause of ill-health but also strongly associated with domestic violence, other crime and high mortality rates. Binge drinking at excessively high to dangerous amounts is higher in many Indigenous populations than non-Indigenous populations in Australia, South America, Canada, Africa and New Zealand (ABS 2006a, Aboriginal Healing Foundation 2003, Steele et al. 2008, Reading and Wein 2009, Montenegro and Stephens 2006, AIHW 2011a, 2011b, Stoner, Stoner and Fryer 2012). Recent rates of hospitalisations and treatments for injuries influenced by excessive binge drinking among Australian and Canadian Aboriginal peoples, American Indian and Alaskan Natives were double that of the national averages in those countries (AIHW 2011a, 2011b, Reading and Wein 2009, US Substance Abuse and Mental Health Services Administration 2010).

Nutrition, physical activity and obesity

Dietary changes among Indigenous peoples across the globe have influenced high rates of disease and illness. By contrast with local traditional foods, many European-introduced foods are often expensive to purchase, lower in nutritional value and high in saturated fats and sugars. The shift away from traditional diets has made a major contribution to high rates of malnutrition and poor health (Langlois, Findlay and Kohen 2013, Plies, Lucas and Ward 2009, AIHW 2011a, Pulver et al. 2010). Low levels of physical activity have compounded these health effects, contributing significantly to higher rates of obesity in many Indigenous communities, including in Canada, the United States and Australia (Casper et al. 2005, Stoner et al. 2012, New Zealand Ministry of Health 2012, AIHW 2008a, Plies et al. 2009, Pulver et al. 2010, Langlois, Findlay and Kohen 2013).

Chronic diseases

The prevalence of chronic illnesses and diseases among Indigenous peoples is the highest in the world (Alderete et al. 1999, Pulver et al. 2010). This contributes to the high mortality rates of many Indigenous peoples, as the following outlines.

TABLE 6.3 *Rates of CVDs among Indigenous compared with non-Indigenous peoples in Australia, Canada and New Zealand, in the years 2005 and 2006*

COUNTRY	INDIGENOUS PEOPLE	RATE OF CVD BY YEAR
Australia	Aboriginal and Torres Strait Islander	1.3 x greater prevalence than non-Indigenous (2005–06)
Canada	All groups	1.5 x greater prevalence than non-Indigenous (2005–06)
New Zealand	Māori	2 x greater mortality than non-Indigenous (2006)

Sources: Compiled from AIHW 2008a, Stoner, Stoner and Fryer 2012, Health Canada 2006, 2009, New Zealand Ministry of Health 2010.

Cardiovascular diseases (CVDs) are among the primary causes of global illness and mortality. As Table 6.3 shows, CVDs are more prevalent and associated with higher rates of mortality among Indigenous peoples in Australia, Canada and New Zealand than their non-Indigenous counterparts (AIHW 2008a, World Heart Federation 2014, Stoner, Stoner and Fryer 2012).

Cancer rates for Indigenous peoples in some countries are largely unavailable due to lack of research in this field. Scant existing data nonetheless show that a large number of Indigenous people die from cancer related to smoking, excessive consumption of alcohol and poor diet or malnutrition. In low-income countries, such as those of sub-Saharan Africa, high cancer mortality rates are more closely related to impaired immune systems attributable to malnutrition and HIV/AIDS (Parkin et al. 2008). But even in wealthy countries, cancer prevalence is on the rise among Indigenous peoples. For example, in 2012, the Canadian Partnership Against Cancer (2011) concluded that cancer was increasing among that country's Indigenous peoples, particularly breast, prostate, lung and colorectal cancers. Cancer in Indigenous populations in Africa, New Zealand, Australia and the Pacific is also rapidly increasing (Sitas et al. 2008, Dachs et al. 2008, AIHW 2013b). In 2006 the rate of cancer deaths among the Māori peoples of New Zealand was already 78 per cent higher than for the non-Māori population (Robson, Purdie and Cormack 2010). Among Indigenous Americans and Alaskan Natives, cancer was the second-highest cause of all deaths in the 2000s (Wiggins et al. 2008). These figures are directly linked to the prevalence of HIV/AIDS, hepatitis and tuberculosis.

Respiratory conditions and infections

Respiratory conditions include asthma, chronic obstructive pulmonary disease (COPD), emphysema and asbestosis. Rates of respiratory conditions are higher among Indigenous peoples than non-Indigenous (see Table 6.4) and correlate directly with rates of 'lifestyle conditions', poor-quality accommodation (such as housing containing asbestos and/or poor insulation) and unsafe workplace health practices (Alderete et al. 1999, Cohen 1999).

Infectious diseases

The *Human Immunodeficiency Virus (HIV)* is a retrovirus that impairs and destroys the immune system, making the infected person more susceptible to infections. According to the WHO (2013e), over 35 million people globally have contracted HIV. Indigenous peoples are identified as one of the most vulnerable groups for HIV infection and transmission (Espinoza et al. 2011). HIV/AIDS is among the biggest causes of ill-health and mortality of Indigenous peoples in sub-Saharan Africa. Its spread is related to the increase of transient labourers and the continuing presence of armed conflict. For example, among the Pygmy people, increasing dependence on participation in employment away from their traditional forest habitat saw the rate of HIV infection increase from nought to 7 per cent between 1993 and 2003 (Ohenjo et al. 2006).

TABLE 6.4 *Rates of respiratory conditions among Indigenous peoples compared with non-Indigenous in Australia, Canada and New Zealand, in the years 2003–08*

COUNTRY (YEAR)	INDIGENOUS PEOPLES	RESPIRATORY CONDITION	RATE
Australia (2003–07)	Aboriginal & Torres Strait Islander	All	Hospitalisation rate is 2–5 x greater than that of all adults over 25 years Prevalence rate is similar for both Indigenous and non-Indigenous
Canada (2003)	First Nations	Chronic bronchitis	Prevalence rate is 1.5 x higher than the national rate
New Zealand (2008)	Māori	COPD	Mortality rate is 3 x greater than the national rate for all adults over 45 years Hospitalisation rate is 4 x greater than the national rate

Sources: Compiled from AIHW 2011a, Health Canada 2009, New Zealand Ministry of Health 2010.

Tuberculosis (TB) is an infectious, bacterial airborne disease that typically affects the lungs and respiratory tract. If not properly treated with appropriate medications, the infection worsens, eventually causing disability or death. It is widely associated with poverty and overcrowded housing (WHO 2013a). Indigenous peoples in countries such as India (Haddad et al. 2012), Canada (Health Canada 2009) and in Latin America (Montenegro and Stephens 2006) have significantly high rates of TB resulting in disablement or death. In some cases, such as in Canada (Health Canada 2009) and African countries (Alderete et al. 1999), TB is a co-infection due to a weakened immune system from malnutrition, pre-existing respiratory conditions or HIV/AIDS.

Mental health

Despite the widespread prevalence of trauma among Indigenous peoples, their mental health is one of the least researched and least understood of all the adverse health conditions they experience. It is nevertheless one of the most debilitating, imposing major barriers to social resources. Psychological trauma is evident in rates of suicide, community and domestic violence and self-harm, which are generally higher in Indigenous communities (Cohen 1999, Oliver, Peters and Kohen 2012, Kochanek et al. 2011). Recent research (Cohen 1999, WHO 2001) demonstrates that racial discrimination (see Chapter 5) is directly linked to mental health conditions, such as depression, psychological trauma and social anxiety, among Indigenous peoples.

Environmental diseases, illness and mortality

Millions of Indigenous peoples have died as a direct result of forced geographic dislocation, often referred to as 'resettlement'. For example, data on the Indigenous peoples of Lao found that their mortality rates doubled as a direct result of forced separation from their traditional homelands (Lao Ministry of Health 2011). In sub-Saharan Africa, high rates of poor oral health (such as tooth decay), intestinal diseases/parasites and viral diseases among Indigenous peoples have been attributed to rapid change in environmental conditions and diets. This situation has been particularly severe in Africa's Equatorial region, which contains the largest area of tropical rainforest on the continent and serves as home to around 300 000 Indigenous hunter–gatherer peoples (Cohen 1999, Ohenjo et al. 2006). Deforestation, logging and dislocation of Indigenous peoples for industrialised farming and global trade have been especially destructive. The dislocation of Pygmy peoples from traditional lands, for example, has resulted in traditional medicines for common health conditions, such as diarrhoea and parasites, becoming scarce or unavailable (Ohenjo et al. 2006, Langlois, Findlay and Kohen 2013). Loss of a forest-based life can be associated with increased mortality. Conversely, Indigenous peoples' experiences of successful land-rights campaigns have been connected with improved mortality. The Twa clan among the Pygmy peoples, for example, experienced improved health soon after they retrieved a proportion of their traditional lands. Mortality in Twa children younger than five years declined from 59 to 18 per cent when their families were given land in their traditional regions (Ohenjo et al. 2006).

A further major source of environmental disease, especially cancer, and of premature mortality among Indigenous peoples, has been the activation of nuclear weapons by foreign powers on or near their land (Cohen 1999, Alderete et al. 1999). From the 1950s to the 1960s, various foreign governments engaged in large-scale nuclear weapon testing programs. 'More than 180 nuclear tests . . . [were] carried out . . . in Polynesia', for example (Alderete et al. 1999: 21). In some countries, Indigenous peoples continue to reside on radioactive soils. Some parts of the Pacific 'depend on food aid because the locally grown food is too radioactive to eat' (Alderete et al. 1999: 21). The environmental hazards for Indigenous peoples in the Pacific region include dumping of hazardous chemical wastes, chemical burn-off, mining, agroforestry and logging (Alderete et al. 1999).

What is the origin of the health division between Indigenous and non-Indigenous peoples?

As we saw in Chapter 2, European modernity developed together with colonisation. The contemporary health division between Indigenous and non-Indigenous peoples documented above originates in this history. One of the clichés that characterises it is that when the first colonisers arrived in the lands of the 'new world', they encountered astonishing riches, including natural abundance. One of them, a 17th-century British lawyer, philosopher and subsequent slave owner called John Locke (1690/1948), described what he witnessed as a 'cornucopia'. This was something that a number of artists of the time used as a symbol of natural abundance – the 'horn of plenty', which was a goat's horn overflowing with flowers, fruit and corn (Oxford English Dictionary 1964: 273). Locke (1690/1948) proposed that what distinguished civilised human beings from 'savages', or those living in a 'state of nature', was private ownership and the development of land and resources. So, when confronted by the cornucopia of the Americas, European colonisers were obliged to seize and develop it in order to pursue their destiny as civilised people. The peoples already inhabiting the lands of plenty were not recognised as 'proper' landowners because they had not appropriated them through individual tenure, nor had they cultivated them for private advancement (Arneil 1994). As a consequence, if they were not killed at the hands of the colonisers, they and their descendants survived as 'Indigenous peoples'.

Locke's 'new world' cornucopia, of course, has been transformed. The wealth of the world's natural abundance and the geographic locations that generate it are now largely in the hands of a fraction of the world's inhabitants, as we saw in Chapter 3. Together with less than one-tenth of the world's 7 billion people, they are the main beneficiaries, although there are enormous disparities, as we have already seen. The contemporary cornucopia owes much of its existence to how the other nine-tenths live; that is, without much at all and in the face of endemic uncertainty. As we have already seen in Chapter 3, the two parts of this global division have been described as the Global North or *metropole* – where the wealthy, powerful and culturally influential minority lives – and the Global South or *periphery* – where the majority is located (Connell 2007: 212–17). Contemporary global division is one of the enduring effects of European colonisation, as is the health inequity between Indigenous and non-Indigenous. The following proposes that while global division perpetuates the divisions between Indigenous and non-Indigenous created by colonisation, it does so through a specific social process – that of *indigeneity*.

Indigeneity: Coercive alienation from land, material resources, language and culture

In proposing that indigeneity is a social process, we are aligning it in a number of ways with its other divisive relatives – class, gender and ethnicity. One of the main features indigeneity shares with these social divisions is *power*; yielding benefits to the dominant at the expense of the subjugated or subordinated.

As a specific domain of social process, however, it is characterised by its own dynamic that produces a distinctive form of inequality and conflict. This dynamic, we suggest, centres on the coercive alienation of colonised peoples from their land, material resources, cultures, languages and law in the name of superior civilisation and human progress. Alienation has many complex meanings (Williams 1976), but central to all of them is the idea of separation. In this chapter we develop a sociological understanding of indigeneity that acknowledges the *separation* of people, both collectively and individually, from control over what were once their lands and material resources, and from social relationships essential to surviving and developing as human beings. Separated in this way, colonised peoples experienced dissolution of the collective identity that underpins social solidarity and cohesion as a people. *Coercive alienation* conveys not only a sense of the physical and social dislocation of such separation, but also of violation and effacement of people as *persons*, similar to what we saw in Chapter 2 with slavery.

As we have seen in relation to previous dynamics of division, indigeneity brings specific *relations of inequality* into being, establishing two main groups of people: Indigenous and non-Indigenous. In the process, they experience hierarchically differentiated access to material, symbolic and agentic resources that are foundational to health. Such a division derives from patterns of practice related to the coercive alienation of colonised peoples from both their lands and material resources, their languages and cultures, and in the name of a superior or 'progressive' humanity. Such structures of practice, then, operate both *materially* and *symbolically*. They do so, however, together with other major dynamics of social division, engendering multiple ways of being and becoming Indigenous. Some sociologists describe the mixing and merging of the various structures of practice related to class, gender, ethnicity and indigeneity, for example, as *intersectionality* (Choo and Ferree 2010). This not only generates diverse cultural experiences of indigeneity but also differentiated access to resources among Indigenous people themselves. The generally small minority of educated, middle-class Indigenous people resident in urban Australia with professional jobs, for example, are much more likely to have better incomes, housing, transportation, nutrition and health care than their unemployed counterparts, who may live in temporary or makeshift accommodation in isolated rural or remote areas, especially in the Northern Territory and Western Australia. Before explaining in greater depth how *indigeneity* gets into peoples' bodies as 'health', the following locates its development within a socio-historical perspective that begins with colonisation and concludes with contemporary global division.

European colonisation and the emergence of indigeneity: Material and symbolic practice

Colonisation is the process by which a social group invades and occupies the traditional lands of another social group, primarily for the purposes of expanding its wealth and power. There have been numerous examples throughout history, including the expansions of the Roman Empire across Western Europe, North Africa and West Asia, the Vikings of Scandinavia into Europe, and the Russian Empire around its neighbouring borders. European colonisation commenced around the turn of the 16th century as Portuguese and Spanish imperial states (see Chapter 7) embarked on their seizure and settlement of much of what are now Central and South America, the West Indies and the south-west of the United States (Wolf 1982). 'By the 1560s there were 40,000 native Americans labouring as slaves in the Brazilian Northeast' (Hemming, cited in Wolf 1982: 134). Around 200 years later, in the late 1700s, the number of the native inhabitants of Peru had declined from 5 million at the time of the Spanish conquest to fewer than 300 000 (Kubler, cited in Wolf 1982: 134). Colonisation was generally accompanied, then, by various strategies for depleting the original inhabitants, including geographic displacement and resettlement, enslavement, introduced diseases and, in some cases, genocide, resulting in the depopulation of thousands of Indigenous communities. Yet, neither the Portuguese nor the Spanish confined their imperial expansion to the Americas. By the early 19th century, together with the Dutch, the French, the Belgians, the Italians and the British, the Spanish had colonised much of the rest of the world. Not that this was a cooperative enterprise. Fierce rivalry and warfare prevailed among the European powers involved because of the competition to possess the spoils and glory of imperial conquest.

European colonisation, however, was neither driven nor enacted simply for material gain. As Chapter 5 explained, European colonisation proceeded on the basis of endemic Eurocentric ideals in which colonised peoples were regarded as less than human. The colonisers conquered, killed and subjugated those whose lands they occupied and annexed in the belief that they, the colonisers, were superior beings – *proper* human beings, not like the 'primitives' they encountered in the Americas, Africa, Asia and the South Pacific. The symbolic universe of the colonisers was every bit as crucial to the project of conquest and appropriation as land and wealth. Driven initially by Christian religious beliefs about their natural superiority (Fredrickson 2002), most believed they were doing 'the natives' a favour by bringing them human progress through European civilisation and Christianity (Hall 2002, 2013). By the 18th century, European colonisers had begun to base their superiority on pseudo-scientific categories and understandings of race, as outlined in the previous chapter. The 'classificatory' work of many authoritative anthropological and ethnographical scientists involved in this process produced hypotheses that Caucasian peoples were the original human race from which the others had diverged or degenerated (Fredrickson 2002). Establishing European mastery over the 'other races' of the world provided an opportunity for them to progress as human beings.

Global division and consolidating indigeneity: Material and symbolic practice

European colonisation established the foundations of contemporary global division. By the end of the 19th century, Europe and North America already commanded much of the world's wealth and were key players in the conflagrations of the first half of the 20th century (Hobsbawm 1987, 1994). The warfare that consumed them basically brought the tensions of 19th century colonialism and imperialism to a spectacular climax, taking several decades (1914–45) to resolve. The contemporary global metropole (Connell 2007) is a kind of phoenix risen from the ashes that settled with the end of the conflicts. Yet, it is no longer a colonising power. Rather, it is a force of global domination that is nourished by a combination of divisive social dynamics such as class, gender and ethnicity. The periphery, as previously mentioned, encompasses most of the rest of the world whose economies and societies are caught up in this politically charged international circuitry. Certainly, their participation yields them dividends – development of industries and infrastructure, employment, tax revenues and so on – but these are slivers of the mother-lode owned and controlled by the Global North. One of the central dynamics is class. As Chapter 3 explained, it is generated by the organisation of production and distribution, and the ownership and control of the resources needed for the process, but it operates both within and between countries – in other words, on a national and global basis. This class dynamic is integral to the global division between the metropole and periphery, and vice versa, but so, too, are other social dynamics, including indigeneity, upon which the global division also acts in shaping. We return to this in the next section.

The global metropole established and maintains its dominance not simply through its expansionary economic activity. According to Raewyn Connell (2007), its metropolitan cultural institutions have been and continue to be critical. Universities, think tanks, museums, art galleries and so on, and the knowledges and forms of representation they produce, are cornerstones of metropolitan superiority. Cultural superiority is achieved in a number of ways, but one of the most powerful is *exclusion from recognition* (see Chapter 3) of those cultural practices and representations that are *not* metropolitan, or are different. Their difference negates them as valuable. According to Edward Said (1978), this process is a European invention that creates an enduring *Other* – the Orient. Said (1978) described the European nations as the Occident and its 'othering' of different peoples and cultures the process of Orientalism. He proposed that the European Other provides an 'image, idea, personality and experience' of European superiority and an ideological framework that legitimises Western science. Orientalism is, therefore, the process by which the Occident deals with the Orient, 'making statements about it, authorising views of it, describing it, teaching it, settling it, ruling over it: in short . . . [it] is a western style for dominating, restructuring and having authority over the Orient' (Said 1978: 3). From Said's theoretical perspective we can understand how symbolic or discursive processes (see Chapter 3), including Western science, continue to contribute to indigeneity and the social inequality that characterises it. As Connell (2007: 7) has commented in relation to the global metropolitan-based social sciences:

> . . . the enormous spectrum of human history that . . . sociologists took as their domain was organised by a central idea: difference between the civilisation of the metropole and other cultures whose main feature was their primitiveness.

The 'Black African', the 'Australian Aboriginal' and the 'American Indian' are examples of metropolitan 'primitives' invented by social scientific discourse, and its contribution to the creation of *global difference*. As the following Australian case study of indigeneity and its effects on health discloses, symbolic difference was just as crucial as the material expropriations involved in colonisation and global division.

Australian Aboriginal and Torres Strait Islander peoples: Indigeneity and health

This case study explains how indigeneity has been enacted and continues to be so in Australia – a part of the Global South, or periphery. It focuses on how the social dynamics of indigeneity get into peoples' bodies as health and structures the analysis around the concept of coercive alienation (introduced above).

Coercive alienation: Land and material resources

The Australian Indigenous population – embracing both Aboriginal and Torres Strait Islander peoples – is now estimated to be 3 per cent of the total population of Australia, numbering around half a million people (AIHW 2013c). Speculative estimates suggest that at the time of the first White settlement in New South Wales in 1788 the number of Aboriginal people in Australia was around 750 000 and the number of languages spoken, 250 (Austin-Broos 2011). There were 'four broad resource regions' (Keen 2004, cited in Austin-Broos 2011: 28): the south-east of Victoria; the south-west of Western Australia; a 'grain belt' from western New South Wales through Central Australia and north to the Kimberley; and a tropical region including Cape York and Arnhem Land. One hundred years later most of coastal and eastern Australia was occupied by White settlers engaged in cattle and sheep grazing, other forms of rural production, timber getting, mining and various industries associated with intensive urban development, including manufacturing, building and construction, retail imports and sales, and so on. Australia was not yet a unified nation. Rather, it was governed as a collection of British colonial outposts. Over that time, hundreds of Indigenous clans and nations along the coast and most of the inland were forced from their lands (Broome 2010, Reynolds 1981, 1996). If they were not killed or did not escape in the process, they were moved into White-managed 'town camps', 'Indigenous reserves' and 'missions'. These residential facilities housed Indigenous peoples from many different territories. For example, in the early 1800s, thousands of Indigenous peoples of Tasmania were rounded up by the British and relocated in Aboriginal missions on the Australian mainland (Ryan 2012).

With the loss of land went traditional food sources and other materials used in the making of equipment, canoes, shelters, medicines, weapons and so on. Over the following 50 years, the remainder of the country that had avoided such settlement became similarly occupied, with Indigenous peoples facing fates comparable to those of their coastal and eastern Australian counterparts. Many were put to work without wages, in return for basic shelter, clothing and food rations – tea, sugar and flour (Anthony 2004, Kidd 2006, Senate Standing Committee on Legal and Constitutional Affairs 2006). Whole industries, such as the cattle industry, developed and thrived on the unpaid labour of Aboriginal stockmen and women (Reynolds 1981, 1996, Broome 2010).

This process, of course, was enacted through bodies. The dispossession of land was bloody and murderous, resulting in many Indigenous communities being annihilated. The colonisers enacted mass killings of Indigenous men, women and children, as Thea Astley's novel (cited at the start of this chapter) discloses. There are now innumerable historical records demonstrating the attempted genocide of the Indigenous peoples. Biomedical warfare was adopted by the British colonisers of Australia (Elder 2003), who intentionally exposed colonised peoples to linen and clothing infected with diseases, such as smallpox and measles. Indigenous women were kidnapped, held hostage and raped. Such behaviour resulted in the spread of sexually transmissible diseases and other infections. The loss of land also produced environmental diseases among Indigenous peoples, insofar as they had to abandon their traditional foods and consume European foods high in refined carbohydrates, especially flour and sugars (Sebastian and Donelly 2013). The loss of land also prevented access to traditional medicines used in treating illnesses and injuries.

As White settlement proceeded, Indigenous peoples resisted the seizure of their land, launching attacks on grazing animals and burning crops (Willmot 1988, Broome 2010). But superior White forces, armed with guns and rifles, subdued most such retaliatory action. In the 1960s, the formation of the Indigenous human rights movement signalled major resistance to the subjugation and marginalisation of Indigenous peoples. Both Indigenous and non-Indigenous peoples across the country protested. One of the most famous protests, the Freedom Rides, was led by Charles Perkins, who drove a bus around urban and rural New South Wales, recording the overt racial discrimination and alienation experienced by Indigenous peoples. The Freedom Rides faced much opposition from many non-Indigenous peoples, especially in a small town called Moree, where the Freedom Riders faced violent aggression from the police and town locals (Guile 2011). Yet, the Freedom Rides contributed to landmark legislative and policy reforms for Indigenous peoples, including the 1967 Referendum, an Australian government proposal to enact change to the Australian Constitution. The result enabled Indigenous peoples to be recognised as Australian citizens. By the early 1970s, the first Indigenous, community managed health organisation was funded in Redfern, New South Wales. The first Indigenous Commonwealth parliamentarian, Neville Bonner, was elected in 1971. At the same time, and persisting into the early 1990s, Indigenous Australians mounted further legal resistance to the alienation of their land through land rights and native title legislation.

Native title is the formal, legal recognition that Indigenous peoples held an interest in property prior to colonial conquest that has survived to this current day, except where it has been extinguished through legislation (Gilbert 2007). Such title acknowledges that Indigenous peoples have a form of responsibility, control or ownership (to put it in European terms) over their lands. Native title, however, is not a simple process favouring Indigenous claimants (O'Brien and Elder 2013). Nevertheless, native title has yielded some success. Around 20 per cent of the country is now officially reclaimed by Indigenous peoples. As many claims continue to be processed by the state (see Chapter 7), this percentage may rise (Bradfield 2005). Some Indigenous peoples are granting leases to corporations for the commercial 'development' of their land, from mining to tourism, and reaping windfall financial dividends as a result. The Arnhem Land Barramundi Fishing Lodge in the Northern Territory is an example of such development. There is also some distribution of mining royalties to communities through the Aboriginal Benefits Account and regional land councils. However, such benefits are concentrated among a small minority of Indigenous peoples, with most excluded from any discernible material advantage (Austin-Broos 2011). Further, Indigenous peoples are increasingly facing claims on their land and material resources by large mining and pastoral corporations that governments support with leasehold arrangements over Indigenous land. In the year after the Australian government passed *The Native Title Amendment (Wik) Act* 1998, restricting native title claims and increasing pastoral leases, there was a doubling in the number of mining leases granted (Northern Territory Department of Primary Industries, Fisheries and Mines 2008).

While Indigenous resistance has focused on land rights and native title for more than 40 years, improved access to other material resources has been modest. In 2008, nearly half of Indigenous households were in the lowest income quintile compared with 5 per cent of non-Indigenous households. Indigenous Australians were three to four times more likely to be unemployed than non-Indigenous peoples (AIHW 2011a). The Australian Institute of Health and Welfare (2011a: 23) stated that 'in 2008, more than one-quarter ... of Indigenous households reported living in dwellings with structural problems, such as major cracks in floors or walls, major electrical/plumbing problems and roof defects.' In addition, Indigenous peoples were four times more likely to be homeless than non-Indigenous peoples (AIHW 2011a). Physical amenity for participation in community and leisure activities is very restricted and poorly maintained (AIHW 2011a).

As recent World Bank (2014f) figures on gross domestic product disclose, the Australian economy is ranked 12 out of 189 countries. It is obviously one of the world's richest countries, with a population of just over 23 million people (ABS 2014). More than 225 years after European settlement, however, it is evident that the supposed 'human progress' justifying the conquest of Indigenous peoples and the seizure of their material resources has not yielded *them* much of the bounty. This ideology – or discourse operating in the interests of some at the expense of the many (Fairclough 1992) – prevails as strongly as it ever has, but in a new form, fine-tuned by the global metropole (see below).

Coercive alienation: Language and culture

The geographic displacement of Australian Indigenous peoples was accompanied by the sudden fragmentation and, in many cases, destruction of traditional cultures and languages. When herded together in missions and camps, Indigenous peoples were forbidden to engage in traditional cultural practices or to speak traditional languages. Many were separated from their clans and thrown together with members of other clans so that communication was very difficult, if not impossible, because of linguistic and cultural differences (Hunter 1993, Reynolds 1996, Kelly et al. 2010, Broome 2010). To hasten the destruction of Aboriginal culture, government policies of assimilation were implemented from the 1800s through to the mid-1900s. Such policies did not encourage intermarriage between Indigenous and non-Indigenous Australians. In fact 'Black–White' unions, or 'miscegenation', as it was called, were considered taboo and were discouraged by Australian governments (Solonec 2013). A tactic deployed by state authorities in implementing assimilation was the forced removal until the 1960s of Aboriginal children from their families and their relocation with White families, especially if they 'looked White'. These children are now known as the Stolen Generations (Australian Human Rights and Equal Opportunity Commission 1997, Kelly et al. 2010).

The violent fracturing of the diverse familial and cultural bonds of Indigenous Australia went hand-in-hand with coercive substitution of the language and cultural practices of British colonisers. This development severed Indigenous Australians from many of the means to develop as people, with trusted social connections through which they could be recognised and valued as belonging. Prior to European settlement, Indigenous peoples' traditional lives were characterised by attachment to place and country, kinship and relatedness, and a specific regional language (Austin-Broos 2011). Material life and ritual life were bound together. Indigenous peoples could only gain access to the symbolic resources of the colonisers if they relinquished their ties to traditional language and culture, complying with what were often abusive and punitive regimes of so-called educational institutions (McLennan and Khavarpour 2004, Dockery 2010, Kelly et al. 2010). In effect, this cultural dislocation amounted to a mass abnegation of Indigenous people as human beings that wrought appalling physical and mental health losses.

The main embodied mechanism by which such devastation happened among many Indigenous Australians was and remains that of severe *trauma*, mentioned at the beginning of this chapter. This 'large-T trauma', as it has been called by some psychologists (see Wallin 2007, cited in Kenny 2013: 193), is an emotional experience of an event that poses a severe threat to a person's security. '[N]atural disasters…war, social dislocation, suffering repeated physical or sexual abuse, actual abandonment, or parental mental illness or severe substance abuse' are the prototypical kinds of events that "cause" 'large-T trauma' (Kenny 2013: 193). It involves injury to parts of the brain that is similar to that of mild traumatic physical injury of the brain, resulting in similar emotional and behavioural effects as depression, anxiety and post-traumatic stress disorder (McAllister and Stein 2010). Repeated psychological trauma in children can produce serious neuronal impairment, inhibiting the development of cognitive and learning capacities. Trauma is deeply implicated in interpersonal relations, particularly in people's capacity to trust and form durable attachments to others (Kenny 2013). The scale of coercive alienation from culture and language among colonised peoples in Australia, then, has meant that trauma has become endemic in some communities, but certainly not all (Kelly et al. 2010). It is re-triggered on a routine basis with continuing loss of family and community members due to high mortality, and through domestic and community violence that are themselves often expressions of trauma. One of the phrases often used to describe this phenomenon is that people 'act out' their trauma against others, especially family members. In situations in which access to material resources is constrained among Indigenous communities (through unemployment, precarious employ-ment, low income, poor housing and so on) such trauma is readily re-ignited.

The health losses associated with alienation from language and culture have been significantly compounded by alienation from the symbolic resources provided by institutionalised education and literacy programs. The forces of educational alienation, often described as institutionalised racism, are complex. Their continuing operation has resulted in only 30 per cent of Indigenous Aus-tralians aged 15–34 years having completed school in 2008, compared to 73 per cent of their non-Indigenous counterparts (ABS 2010). There has been some improvement since then but Indigenous and non-Indigenous rates continute to disclose significant disparity.

> In 2013, the national…retention rate for Aboriginal and Torres Strait Islander students from Year 7/8 to Year 12 was 55.1%. This has increased by 16.0 percentage points since 2003 when it was 39.1%. Despite this increase, the rate remains 27.8 percentage points behind the equivalent national rate for all other students in 2013 (82.9%). (ABS 2013b)

This schooling participation profile has been accompanied by Indigenous lit-eracy rates that are among the worst in the world (AIHW 2011a, Department of Prime Minister and Cabinet 2014). Accordingly, Indigenous alienation from institutionalised educational resources has imposed serious constraints on access to further training, jobs and adequate incomes. Low education and training, and high unemployment, both of which are connected to drug and alcohol abuse (Weatherburn 2014), are strongly implicated in imprisonment rates of Indigenous Australians – widely regarded as one of the most overt practices of institutionalised racism. In 2013, more than a quarter (27 per cent) of all Australian prisoners (ABS 2013a), and 86 per cent of those in Northern Territory prisons, identified as Indigenous.

An expression of Indigenous peoples' resistance to colonisation is the return by many to traditional cultural lifestyles. For example, in the Northern Territory and parts of adjoining states, some Indigenous people have returned to a 'traditional lifestyle' through the Homelands Movement (House of Representatives Standing Committee on Aboriginal Affairs 1987). This involves living at 'outstations' on traditional land in traditional shelters, hunting and gathering food, participating in traditional ceremonies and speaking a regional language, among other things. Many are engaged in environmental management through culling of wildlife and the production of fine arts and crafts (Altman 2001). Durable social benefits are reported to result from this movement for Indigenous peoples and the local envi-ronments, but some point to low rates of participation in education, poor literacy levels in children and young people, and limited opportunities for employment as significant costs (Austin-Broos 2011). There is, however, evidence that the Homelands Movement has produced significantly improved health conditions in *some* Indigenous communities that are strongly associated with 'cultural and natural resources management' (Burgess et al. 2005, Garnett and Sithole 2007).

Coercive alienation in the name of civilisation and progress

As previously explained, European colonisation proceeded in the belief that Europeans and their Christian civilisation were superior to the peoples whose lands they expropriated and whose lives they destroyed. By the 18th century, this racist superiority began to incorporate a new ideological dimension: Europeans and their civilisation were increasingly understood as representing a form of human progress that would result in the betterment of everybody (Williams 1976). It was considered that the spread of industrialised production and its work disciplines, scientific classification and rationality, European art and music, centralised and bureaucratic governance, and Christian morals would civilise and transform the world, putting an end to 'savages' and 'savagery'. The symbolic or representational realm of European colonisation, and its absolute certainty about the superiority of its civilisation and the rightness of its mission, was critical in enabling Europeans to treat the original inhabitants of the lands they occupied in the ways they did. This is expressed in the following extract from a novel, set in colonial Tasmania, by the Australian author Richard Flanagan (2008). The Protector of Aboriginal children in Hobart Town has been asked to deliver Mathinna, a 12-year-old Aboriginal orphan, to the Governor and his wife, Lady Jayne Franklin, who are childless.

Tasmania, Australia, late 1830s

Of the children of Ham that had not perished, she [Mathinna] was the brightest...and...perhaps the one with the greatest possibility of [Christian] redemption.

[T]he protector was loathe to part with...Mathinna [but] he told himself, it was to the very finest flowers of England, disciplined in habit, religious in thought, scientific in outlook -- a woman who seemed to be the worthy consort of a man celebrated as one of the greatest names in the annals of heroic endurance, and that man himself [that he was sending the child]. And their selfless goal? To raise the savage child to the level of a civilised Englishwoman. How could he deny anyone such opportunity? (Flanagan 2008: 110--11)

The sense of cultural superiority established through colonisation continues with global division, but it is based on the idea that the economies and democracies of Europe and North America are the epitome of contemporary human progress (Tully 2012). Economic growth and capital accumulation are understood to be the foundations of such progress. Pre-eminent global metropolitan institutions that represent themselves as champions of *global* interests, such as the World Bank, identify and understand global poverty – and the marginalisation of Indigenous peoples – essentially as failures in economic growth – usually called 'under-development'. They subscribe to and propagate a global metropolitan economic orthodoxy that under-development can only be properly redressed through economic growth and the 'trickle-down' effect (Stiglitz 2000). It is a matter of making the economic cake bigger, not distributing the slices of the prevailing one more equitably. Yet, 'the evidence *against* [emphasis added] trickle-down economics is overwhelming' (Stiglitz 2008: 68). This economic ideology is central to the ways in which the corporations and state institutions of the global metropole are able to continue to ignore the material and social effects of indigeneity and all the processes of social division, in fact. Basically, Indigenous peoples are understood as failing *themselves* if they persist with their traditional ways of doing things. They must engage in contemporary human progress by participating in and building market economies.

Conclusions

Contemporary indigeneity is a major social dynamic responsible for Indigenous peoples' experiences of health and health care. Specific to it – and by contrast with class, gender and ethnicity – is the establishment of social inequality through European colonisation and global division. This process centres on seizure of colonised peoples' land and material resources, and the destruction of their languages and cultures, in the name of superior civilisation and human progress. At the heart of the process, from a sociological perspective, is coercive alienation, central to which is the enactment of power through domination/ subjugation *and* resistance between Indigenous and non-Indigenous peoples. Its effects circulate in embodied ways, with subjugation generating health experiences and outcomes that are among the worst in the world.

Indigeneity began on the basis of Eurocentric beliefs and understandings that were predominantly Christian and pseudo-scientific, and situated in the metropole. The metropole perceived the colonised inhabitants as inferior, primitive peoples who were not deserving of the human rights of civilisation. Such a process was inherently discursive, in the sense that it controlled the naming, claiming and understanding of things – the symbolic realm – including the identities of the peoples subjected to the material violence that characterised it (Fanon 1966, 1967). Indigenisation continues as alienation of colonised peoples' lands and cultures proceeds in the name of advanced civilisation and progress, characterised by economic growth, the application of Western scientific knowledges and modes of governance that emanate from the global metropole.

The experience of indigeneity in Australia reflects the invasive and destructive effects of European colonisation and their consolidation through global division. The diversity of Indigenous peoples means that this experience is not 'all of a piece', but many have shared its irreparable damage. By using Australia as a case study, we have demonstrated the magnitude of Indigenous peoples' suffering and the quantifiable health effects from the embodied reverberations of systematic violence, exclusion and marginalisation. Organised resistance, however, has challenged Indigenous peoples' alienation on a number of fronts and with significant successes, including the franchise and land rights. Measurable health outcomes reveal significant improvements in some areas but advocates of global metropolitan progress insist that further advancement depends on participation in commercial development and labour markets. Remnant traditions of northern Australian indigeneity are not so convinced as they sculpt new ways of living on and within the boundaries of markets to progress Aboriginal 'body, land and spirit' (Reid 1982).

Questions for discussion

1 What was European colonisation?
2 What is global division?
3 From a sociological perspective, what do you understand by the term 'coercive alienation' in relation to indigeneity and Indigenous peoples?
4 How can indigeneity be understood as a social dynamic or process?
5 What does it mean to describe Indigenous health as the combination of embodied effects of indigeneity?
6 What health evidence outlined in the 'snapshots' in this chapter provide strong empirical bases for the proposal that coercive alienation has caused higher rates of morbidity, mortality and disability among Indigenous peoples? Explain your choice.

7 What do you think have been the most damaging material and symbolic dimensions of indigeneity in the Australian context for Indigenous peoples?

8 How have Indigenous Australians resisted alienation and its effects?

9 How can economic growth and market-based interventions be understood as human progress? Do they offer any solutions to the problem of health inequity arising from indigeneity?

7 The state and health

Toni Schofield and Marco Berti

Overview

- What is 'the state'?

- How did rationalised rule and governance differ from their predecessors? What role did they play in the development of democratic states?

- What is neo-liberalism and what are the main processes by which it is played out in contemporary rule and governance? How do these affect health inequity?

- What is the relationship between the state and other major processes of social division?

- How do contemporary rule and governance establish barriers to and opportunities for the advancement of health equity?

Timor-Leste (East Timor)

To the north of Australia lies the 21st century's first nation state – Timor-Leste, or East Timor. After a period of brutal control by Indonesia, which had taken over the former Portuguese colony in 1975, Timor-Leste formally gained its independence in 2002. Today, Timor-Leste is one of Asia's poorest countries, with more than 80 per cent of its 1.2 million people resident in rural areas. Yet, it has become one of the fastest-growing countries in the world, with a national budget of over US $1 billion per year. Its newfound wealth derives from vast stores of oil and gas in the Timor Sea that have been used to establish a government fund estimated to be worth close to US $12 billion dollars. Along with this wealth has emerged a major rift about what the government should spend this money on.

To date, the Timor-Leste government has prioritised infrastructure projects – such as construction of a national power grid and power plant, roads and bridges – and improved pension payments for older people and veterans, among a variety of other favoured concerns. However, members of the Opposition and other critics say that spending should concentrate on the country's human development, by improving education, health care and agricultural irrigation, especially since the overwhelming majority of Timor-Leste's people are subsistence farmers. With poverty rates above 40 per cent, the world's third-highest rate of child malnutrition, widespread infectious disease and a fertility rate that matches global leaders – sub-Saharan Africa and Afghanistan – Timor-Leste faces health challenges that are among the world's toughest.

One of the main mechanisms that countries in the Global South have for addressing the formidable health challenges they face is government action through public policy and funding. In East Timor, there is obvious conflict about whether the government should prioritise funding of health-related measures over other concerns. Government policies, and the public debates and discussions that characterise them, have a major bearing on people's health, as this chapter explores in detail. However, government policies and public discussions are part of a broader social process that we call 'the state'; a concept introduced in Chapter 2. This chapter re-visits the state, providing more in-depth explanation of what it is, how it works and how it plays a central role in determining social inequalities and health inequities. While the state is in bad repute in some quarters – with pejorative media references to 'totalitarian states', 'rogue states', 'lawless states' and 'nanny states' – the state's effect on global health renders it critical in terms of intervening in health equity. Before examining its contemporary operation and effects on health, we turn first to how the state emerged historically.

The emergence of the state

The state is a specific domain of social process that involves the exercise of centralised authority. It is widely regarded as the epicentre of organised political activity, both within and between countries. *What distinguishes the state as a social process from others, such as class, gender, ethnicity and indigeneity, is its exercise of rule and governance.* Some suggest that the state's operation is so important that without it society would collapse – an idea first espoused by the English philosopher Thomas Hobbes (Schmitt 2008). Subsequently, some historians and social scientists have argued persuasively that most contemporary societies owe their very existence to the state (see, for example, Hobsbawm 1994, Connell and Dados 2014). The state and centralised governance, however, are comparatively recent social creations, as the following explains.

Anatomically modern humans have inhabited Earth for at least 200 000 years, but for 98 per cent of this time (Carneiro 1994) they lived in small bands without centralised governance. Life was based on hunting and gathering (Claessen and Skalnik 1978), and simple divisions of labour (see Chapter 2) related to gender and age. For example, the work of hunting was mainly undertaken by men, and gathering by women (Dahlberg 1981). The first examples of centralised organisations that ruled over peoples only emerged after the agricultural revolution, with the introduction of agricultural production and animal husbandry over 10 000 years ago. The growth of dense populations that ensued triggered the establishment of rule and control, accompanied by specialised governance. This development is estimated to have occurred around 6000 years ago (Diamond 2012). Settled agriculture and pastoralism revolutionised human life. It made the production of large food surpluses more reliable and provided a foundation for the release of a minority of people from having to participate in subsistence farming and to engage in other activities, such as governance. The 'selection process' – that is, the grounds on which some got to be rulers and the methods by which they secured their position – remains obscure. Yet, it is evident that governance brought with it a new social hierarchy: between the rulers and the ruled. Once installed, rulers mobilised a range of measures to maintain their privilege and power, and its transmission to subsequent family members. The compulsory collection of taxes from the ruler's subjects was one of the key mechanisms. This was enforced by the ruler's control over the means of violence or force – usually an army or police force – supported by the collection of taxes (Elias 1994). Purported links with deities and the divine were also commonly used by rulers to justify their power and privilege. These alleged connections were routinely reinforced by religious organisations and those designated to uphold and oversee their beliefs and practices, such as the Catholic clergy in pre-modern Europe.

Governance in pre-medieval European states was widely characterised by capricious decisions made by monarchs or local warlords who often were supported by an inner circle or council that acted as a kind of advisory body. Members of these assemblies exercised considerable power because they often served the sovereign as successful warriors, controlling large areas of the royal domain. In many such places, only they were authorised to collect the levies and taxes upon which the sovereign relied (Luiten van Zanden, Buringh and Bosker 2010). By 1200–1500, many of these councils became more formalised and independent, establishing *parliaments* that actively constrained the absolute and frequently tyrannical rule of European monarchs (Luiten van Zanden, Buringh and Bosker 2010). These initially comprised members of the nobility (feudal lords), the Church (bishops) and the medieval cities (mayors and rich merchants). They *represented* the 'subjects of the (sovereign's) realm' (Luiten van Zanden, Buringh and Bosker 2010: 6), coming together to discuss their *interest*s (Williams 1976), as they understood them. The consent of a king or queen was an essential requirement for these medieval parliaments but they nevertheless acted as significant constraints on monarchical power. Their main functions were the granting of taxes proposed by the sovereign, participation in law making and decisions on war and peace, appointment or abdication of a sovereign, and even serving on high courts of justice (Marongiu 1968, cited in Luiten van Zanden, Buringh and Bosker 2010).

Still, by the 1600s, it was the network of monarchs and their aristocratic relatives that formed the centre of European governance. So much so that the state was typically considered the private embodiment of monarchs – an idea epitomised by Louis XIV's famous statement: 'I am the State'. However, managing a large territory with a big population demanded more than what one person and his or her immediate entourage could do on their own. Administering power in this situation generated an organisational mechanism called *bureaucracy*. While its original introduction 'stretches back into antiquity, especially the Confucian bureaucracy of the Han dynasty… [its modern form] emerged in France in the eighteenth century' (Clegg 2007: 376). This innovation offered much tighter control and accountability of those designated by royal sovereigns to manage their wealth, and freed them from their reliance on local taxes over which parliaments had some say (Luiten van Zanden, Buringh and Bosker 2010).

The sovereigns of these early European states typically regarded people's health in instrumental terms; that is, as a resource for maintaining their rule. Healthy subjects were more productive. They could pay more taxes and fight in the ruler's armies, protecting or expanding territorial borders as required. As significantly, they could bear children more reliably, ensuring supply of labour and taxes. As a consequence rulers were only concerned with the collective health of the populace, not that of individuals, as their responses to epidemics made apparent. With the spread of plague in late medieval Europe, for example, monarchs focused on controlling the movements of the sick and infected by means of quarantine regulations and limitations on trade, travel and gatherings of people (Slack 1988). The actual provision of care for sick and dying people was not a ruler's responsibility. This fell to local villagers, usually women – 'wisewomen and midwives' (Ehrenreich and English 1979) – and the medieval Church that established and ran the early European 'hospitals' (Foucault 1976, Rosen 1963).

Nation states

The pre-modern European state disappeared with the rise of nations and nationalism that began in the 16th century as imperial Spain embarked on its colonisation of South America (Fitzpatrick 2001). The modern state, then, developed through 'nation building' that went hand-in-hand with European colonialism (Hobsbawm 1992). Bloody and conflicted, this project involved countless wars between and among European powers, throughout which they planted their models of governance among those whom they colonised. The spread of European rule, however, did not necessarily mean the imposition of centralised authority among 'state-less', so-called 'primitive peoples', as discussed in Chapter 6. Colonising powers were often forced to work with powerful and well-established local regimes, such as those that prevailed in imperial China and India (see, for example, Mitra 2005, Swamy 2011), creating new forms of governance in the process (Connell and Dados 2014).

Nowadays, the current geographic pervasiveness of nation states makes them 'the most dominant geopolitical unit the world has ever known' (Penrose and Mole 2008: 271). The only areas of the planet that are not considered legal property of any state are uninhabitable portions of Antarctica and seas more than 200 nautical miles offshore (Brilmayer and Klein 2001). It is the exclusive control over a clearly defined and delimited territory that is a distinctive feature of contemporary nation states – a development inextricably linked to the advancement of mapping technologies that were a crucial feature of modernising and colonising Europe (Branch 2011). Today, despite their different geographic and social locations, their sizes and histories, nation states display remarkable similarities in the ways in which they work. They use standardised ways of counting and classifying their citizens; they organise their administration around ministries and agencies; and they extract taxes and regulate economic behaviours. This similarity derives in large measure from the global permeation of *modern rationality,* which we discuss more fully below. It accompanied colonisation and the dominance of the European metropole throughout the world.

Rationalised governance and the modern state

Early modern European states faced complex and diverse challenges with the effects of industrialisation and colonialism (see Chapters 2 and 6). Widespread crime, riots, contagious diseases, contaminated water supply, wars and colonial uprisings, rapid proliferation in trade and investment, and the mass exodus and influx of people across Europe, for example, posed major threats to European stability. They challenged the conditions needed for generating profits and ac-cumulating private property, and the steady production and distribution of goods and services on which they depended. The modern state emerged largely in response to these developments, irrevocably changing the foundations of governance.

According to German sociologist Max Weber (1930/1974), this new approach to governance was symptomatic of a broader social transformation that he called *rationalisation.* This process marked a major departure from pre-modern European life and the prevalence of belief in magic, mystery and the inexplicable. At the heart of rationalisation lay a preoccupation with the *utility* of things, goal-oriented activity and the replacement of concern about quality with relentless calculation and measurement of quantity (Beilharz 1991). For Weber (1930/1974), rationalisation was what enabled the capitalist accumulation of profits, distinguishing industrialised capitalism from its historical predecessors. It operated primarily through tight controls over the organisation of work and production (see Chapter 3). The aim of rationalising *governance* was to achieve consistency and predictability that would foster investment and commerce, protecting and advancing the 'wealth of the nation' (Williams 1976: 280–1). The main instrument by which rationalised governance was established was *bureaucratisation.* Already embedded in the work of European production by the mid-19th century, as Weber explained, it permeated the administrative apparatus of governance. In 19th-century Europe, bureaucracy was designed to control the actions of everybody who participated in it and ensure delivery of the goals specified by their masters. This was achieved through an hierarchical chain of command. Written and impersonal rules that prescribed standardised, impartial and uniform administrative decisions and actions were to apply to everyone equally and fairly. In other words, nobody could expect preferential treatment because of his or her privileged birth or connections with the administrators or their rulers. With 19th-century bureaucratisation, modern administration was undertaken by professional bureaucrats; that is, civil servants, or *officials* (Weber 1930/1974) who did not own their offices but temporarily occupied them. These administrators were selected on the basis of *merit*, demonstrated through qualifications for the job, which sometimes involved competitive public examinations. Such a selection process was instituted to prevent bias and nepotism in the appointment of state officials and corruption in public administration, securing *legitimacy* of administrative governance.

The legitimate rule over people emerged as a major source of conflict and civil war in Europe in the 17th century, especially in Britain. Monarchical governance provoked violent opposition because of its autocratic power, and parliaments became independent of sovereigns (Luiten van Zanden, Buringh and Bosker 2010). In Britain these parliaments consisted of assemblies of 'the people' who elected them (Aron 1965). They worked as institutions of representative governance. *Popular consent* was demanded as the foundation of legitimate governance (Locke 1690/1948). By the 19th century, alongside the rationalisation of administration, parliaments occupied a central place in modern governance, discussing and formulating goals and rules, or *policies* and *laws*. Yet, until the latter half of the 19th century, those whom parliaments represented were only a tiny minority of 'the people', usually wealthy landowning men. This pattern of representation prevailed also in British colonial parliaments, such as that of New South Wales in Australia. Parliamentary representatives participated in this process along collectively oppositional lines, in the manner of the Tories and the Whigs of the British Parliament. The basis for *suffrage*, or the *right* to elect representatives in the parliament, was vigorously challenged by other constituencies throughout the 19th century, with the ownership of property and masculine gender abolished as requirements for participation (Hobsbawm 1969a). While parliaments discussed and debated policies and laws, it was *governments* – not monarchs – that decided what they were to be, and how they were to be implemented. The bureaucracy, through its network of departments and public agencies, was responsible for administering and implementing government decisions. Determining the lawfulness of the rules, settling disputes arising in the course of their implementation, and punishing those who transgressed them remained the responsibility of the judiciary and court system. The police and armed forces operated to enforce parliamentary and judicial decisions.

These social processes and their combined interaction on a day-to-day basis played an integral role in a system of modern European governance that eventually terminated monarchical rule, if not the monarchs themselves. So began modern *electoral representative democracy* (Williams 1976). Not that such a process evolved rationally and consensually. Crucial to the development of democratised governance was organised and often violent struggle by those who historically had been excluded from 'the people' – that is, those authorised to vote for representation in parliament. By 1973, representative democratic governance had spread to 45 of the world's 151 countries and increased by the late 1990s to 120 countries, or more than 60 per cent of the world's independent states (Fukuyama 2011). The democratic state not only demands abolition of the division between rulers and ruled but also a commitment in the practice of governance to serve the interests of all of the nation's citizens – the *public* or *general good* (Mill 1910/1972). The democratic state as a legitimate form of governance must ensure *popular sovereignty*, or the will of the people in the exercise of its rule (Locke 1690/1948). One of the main instruments by which it is expected to do so is rationalisation. Though democratic rule by its very nature incorporates popular preferences in framing and implementing policies and laws, it is nevertheless expected to transcend 'narrow' or 'sectional' interests through the application of rules and procedures that show no favour to any particular group (Schumpeter 1943/1987). Further, while parliamentary debate and government decisions are supposed to canvas the diverse spectrum of values and priorities, they are also required to be informed and guided by expert technical – and therefore, impartial – advice (Wilenski 1987, Yeatman 1990). All this is expected to be conducted in accordance with a constitution, or the written rules embodying the aspirations and interests of the nation's citizenry. The state in contemporary democratic societies, then, is widely proposed to operate as a *neutral umpire* negotiating diverse and conflicting interests but making and enforcing decisions that express the collective will and optimise the public good.

Neo-liberalism, state dynamics and health inequity

The rationalisation and democratisation of governance have made dramatic progress on a global basis, especially over the past 40 years, but their effect on health inequity, both within and between countries, has been modest to say the least. In fact, despite its proclaimed neutrality, the modern democratic state in capitalist societies plays a robustly partisan political role (see, for example, Fraser 1989, Offe 1996, Tully 2012). As the following outlines, there are a number of processes by which contemporary states operate that consistently generate social inequality and health inequity. This trend has in fact intensified with the development of what social scientists have called *neo-liberalism* (Connell and Dados 2014, Dean 2014, Harvey 2005, 2010). On the one hand, this can be understood as a particular patterning or structure in the practices of governance and rule. On the other hand, it is also one of the world's most influential approaches to the operation of states. It is informed by an international movement that has adopted thinking that can be called a 'thought collective' (Dean 2014: 151–3). At the heart of this thinking is that universal wealth and well-being can best be achieved by embracing competition, promoting business and markets, and providing an institutional framework that safeguards private property rights, free trade and economic growth (Harvey 2005). Neo-liberalism can also be understood in terms of what it opposes – primarily economic protection, state intervention in the market and 'mass social programs' (Dean 2014: 151–2), including education, healthcare and welfare. Neo-liberalism is connected to the expansion and influence of large corporations and their power over nation states and democratic governance (see Chapter 3) (Fuchs 2007, Connell and Dados 2014).

The following outlines and discusses the main state processes involved in the production and contestation of social inequality and health inequity, both within and between countries. These are: i) regulation and deregulation, ii) re-distribution (taxes and transfers), iii) corporatisation and marketisation, iv) individualisation, and v) participation (marginalisation/exclusion). Social inequality and health inequity have not been deliberate goals of these processes. In some notable cases, especially regulation and re-distribution, they have actually advanced social equality and health equity. State processes per se, then, do not necessarily enact and support dominant political interests associated with class, gender, ethnicity and indigeneity. Yet, the latter play a powerful role in shaping state processes and, as a consequence, impose formidable limits on what states can do in intervening in social inequality. In fact, rule and governance, and the dynamics of social division, work as a two-way street. The processes of the state *interact* with those of class, gender, ethnicity and indigeneity.

Regulation and health equity

Regulation is one of the mechanisms by which the state is distinguished from other domains of social practice. It is a social process of restriction or control, enacted through the formulation of laws and policies, and their implementation by the courts, police and other public sector agencies. The central aims of regulation are to prevent some social practices while encouraging others. One of the major consequences of this process is the establishment of legally enforceable *rights*. These operate as institutionalised means by which individuals and collectives can have their claims to resources recognised and acted upon. Regulation has been around since the establishment of centralised governments in various forms, but contemporary 'prototypes' were crafted in the 19th century with the rise of industrialisation (see Chapter 2). The Factory Acts legislated by the British Parliament between 1833 and 1864 (Doyal and Pennell 1979), for example, were among the first to regulate and control employment and working conditions. These acts reduced the working day to 10 hours and forbade the employment of women and children in industries in which they competed with men (Barrett and McIntosh 1982, Walby 1986), an issue previously discussed in relation to gender dynamics (see Chapter 4). The first of these acts provided for four inspectors and eight sub-inspectors 'with authority to fine offenders on the spot and other extensive enforcement powers' (Bartrip and Burman 1983: 18). In the face of the depth and breadth of the barbarity of British factory employment at the time, the number of inspectors appointed meant that effective enforcement was minimal. However, the Act did establish the principle of inspection as a means of enforcing legislation more broadly.

Lord Althorp, the Factory Acts and health

The first of the Factory Acts and the provision to appoint inspectors was based on a bill introduced by the Chancellor of the Exchequer, Lord Althorp, who energetically resisted any specific provision for 'industrial health and safety'. By the early 19th century, industrial injuries and deaths were a serious issue causing incalculable misery to working people, especially in the textile mills and coal mines. As the Factories Inquiry Commission of 1833 reported, 'the danger of being killed or injured by a machine...was "one of the great evils to which people employed in factories are exposed"' (Bartrip and Burman 1983: 12). However, when the Commission's report was presented in Parliament, Lord Althorp protested that any bills to prevent industrial accidents and to provide compensation were 'unjust' and would be 'disastrous in the manufacturing districts' (Bartrip and Burman 1983: 17). Lord Althorp's opposition was vigorously supported by many, both inside and outside the Parliament. William Hylett MP commented that punishment of a proprietor for a death arising from a machine accident was improper because this was a 'comparatively small offence' for which the proprietor might not be to blame at all (Bartrip and Burman 1983: 17–18). A Scottish manufacturer wrote, 'I have no hesitation in saying that if passed...[industrial safety legislation] would be utterly impracticable for any man to conduct an establishment where machinery is used' (Bartrip and Burman 1983: 18). The industrial safety question was consigned to oblivion until further parliamentary investigations recommenced in 1840, eventually leading to the Factory Act 1844. It was this legislation that introduced the first provisions for forcing employers to comply with very minimal safety regulation and the possibility of an employer fine if an injured worker could successfully demonstrate in court that injury had incurred due to workplace machinery that had been inadequately guarded.

As the above case study shows, early economic regulation involving modest provisions to improve the health of working people in Britain struck at the heart of the relations between workers and employers – or labour and capital. As Lord Althorp and his supporters disclosed, it was unacceptable because it represented an attack on the wealth and privilege of the dominant class. Being forced to put guards around dangerous machinery would slow down production and eat into profits. As significantly, introducing legislation and possible fines on employers to prevent workplace deaths and injuries was an assault on what they saw as their private property and their right to use and manage it in ways they deemed fit. Since then, 'workplace health and safety' (WHS) regulation has advanced across the Global North, with major improvements in working people's health (ILO 2005). It is one of the central mechanisms by which the state has been an active player in reducing the disparity in health between owners/controllers of the production and distribution of goods and services, and the resources needed for the process, and those who do the work involved.

Much of the global burden of workplace death and injury has been transferred to the 'developing world' – especially China, South Asia and South-east Asia (see Hamalainen, Saarela and Takala 2009) – where WHS regulation reflects approaches that prevailed in 19th-century Britain.

There are many other forms of state regulation that influence social inequality and health inequity. Despite the rise of neo-liberalism and its opposition to market regulation, there is still significant regulatory governance that controls potentially harmful market-based activities. Such a process offers the greatest benefits to those with the least resources because the onus of redress for harms or damage caused by the sale of products and services lies with state agencies rather than individual consumers. *Individual responsibility* for market-based harms and costs places the greatest burden on those with the least resources (see below). Building regulations that aim to control unsafe and damaging housing and other construction, for example, place the responsibility for faults and defects that can cause harm to their occupants on those who produce and sell them. These regulations enforce responsibility through the threat of public prosecution through the court system for failure to comply. Like many other similar regulations related to the production of goods and services, they limit health inequity because individuals are not held fully responsible for protecting themselves from damages caused by the purchase of faulty products. Food regulations focusing on hygienic production and distribution to prevent food poisoning and other health hazards further illustrate the point, as does the regulation of nursing homes and institutional care. In relation to the latter, state regulation is designed to support more vulnerable constituencies, such as frail older people and people with disabilities, in finding accommodation and care that does not exploit and harm them.

Regulation of wages and conditions is also a form of market control – namely, the labour market. Such regulation protects working people from a variety of employment-related harms. It imposes limits on the extent to which employers can exploit the labour they hire, especially by restricting the amount of hours and times employers can expect workers to work, and the surplus they can extract as profits (see Chapters 2 and 3). For example, in most high-income countries at least, employment legislation specifies and enforces minimum wages, the number of hours full-time employees can be expected to work on a weekly basis, and compulsory paid leave entitlements. Through such regulation employers are prevented from forcing workers to participate in arrangements and conditions of employment that cause them – and often their families – harm or distress. Such restrictions have been critical in improving 'social standards of living' (McKinlay and McKinlay 2009) and in contributing to advancing health equity – at least in the countries of the rich world. Despite such a contribution, further improvements in these conditions, such as increasing the minimum wage, are typically opposed by business and employer groups that claim they have adverse financial and employment effects. There is no evidence, however, of such a relationship in most OECD countries (Oliver and Buchanan 2014).

Deregulation: Workplace and environmental health effects and inequities

State enthusiasm for regulatory processes, however, especially in the Anglo-democracies, has been waning with the spread of neo-liberal governance. Governments and their advisers have supported growing deregulation of certain areas of goods and service production and distribution and the ownership or control of the resources needed for the process. Deregulation involves the removal of laws and other controls, mainly over business, purportedly to improve market efficiency and to reduce government and bureaucratic costs associated with regulation.

War on 'red tape', Australia 2014

In Australia, the Liberal–National Coalition Government is embarking on a massive program of deregulation and cutting of 'red tape'. The government has promised to cut $1 billion in red tape annually, repealing more than 8000 regulations and laws considered redundant. The red tape reduction bill is designed to reduce the volume of regulation, eliminate duplication between state and federal governments, improve consultation with business and ensure greater transparency and efficiency within the public service. According to the Prime Minister's parliamentary secretary for deregulation, 'all cabinet submissions that have a major regulatory impact will now be subject to a regulatory impact statement and all senior ministers are required to establish a deregulation unit within their department' (Massola 2014).

There is no evidence, however, that deregulation makes any significant contribution to improved health. In fact, the *absence* of state regulation is widely associated – indeed, considered a direct cause of – major illness, injury and fatality affecting mainly those who are already struggling to survive as a result of the dynamics of social inequality. For example, the collapse of the Rana

Plaza factory in Bangladesh in 2013, which killed 129 garment workers, almost all women, has revealed an astonishingly laissez-faire approach. This basically means that the state is prepared to let business get on with doing what it wants, clearly demonstrated in Bangladesh's building and construction industries, employment conditions, and workplace health and safety (ILO 2014). Their combination has made Bangladesh a highly attractive destination for invest-ment by manufacturers from the Global North. While there is long-established state regulation of workplace deaths and injuries in Australia, recent develop-ments suggest that public sector agencies responsible for this work are relin-quishing the use of their coercive powers to promote employers' compliance with workplace health and safety laws in favour of 'softer', educational and advisory interventions (Schofield, Reeve and McCallum 2014). Such a direction is indicative of the increasing deregulation of the Australian economy and a regulatory approach in which business can grow and prosper at the expense of the 'public good' (Rees, Rodley and Stilwell 1993). Such an approach, of course, is not confined to Australia. It is intrinsic to neo-liberal governance, deepening inequality across the globe (Stiglitz and Lin-Yifu 2014).

The absence of regulation or presence of minimal regulation related to 'physical threats to the environment' (Baum 2008: 309) is a further exam-ple illustrating the state's active contribution to health damage and inequity. The main physical threats to the environment affect the Earth's atmosphere and climate, and the quality of air, water and soil. In respect to the former, the burning of fossil fuels, carbon emissions and ozone-depleting gases pose the main threats through their effects on global warming and climate change (Flannery 2005). As results of global attempts to control 'greenhouse gas' emis-sions disclose, however, regulation of the threats involved is extremely limited (Baum 2008). The effects on people's health have already commenced and are anticipated to have dramatic future effects on global health through climate change, as the recent report by the United Nation's Intergovernmental Panel on Climate Change (IPCC 2014) discloses.

The Intergovernmental Panel on Climate Change (IPCC 2014)

How does climate change affect human health?
According to the IPCC, climate change affects health: i) through the mortality and morbidity (including 'heat exhaustion') arising from extreme heat events, floods and other catastrophic weather events in which climate change may play a role; ii) from environmental and ecosystem changes that create direct

effects, 'such as shifts in patterns of disease-carrying mosquitoes and ticks, or increases in waterborne diseases due to warmer conditions and increased precipitation and runoff' (IPCC 2014: 36); and
iii) indirectly through such conditions as hunger and food insecurity arising from reduced agricultural production; stress, mental illness and violent conflict caused by population displacement; financial strains and losses from declining productivity arising from the effects of heat exhaustion on the workforce, or other enrionmental stressors; and 'damage to health care systems by extreme weather events' (IPCC 2014: 37).

Who is most affected by climate change?
Those with 'existing disease burdens... with the weakest health protection systems, and with least capacity to adapt' (IPCC 2014: 37) will be most adversely affected by climate change. So, as most of the reputable assessments suggest, in general it will be the poor and disenfranchised who will suffer the highest risk. On a global basis, poor countries will incur the greatest burden, especially their millions of impoverished children, 'who are most affected by such climate-related diseases as malaria, undernutrition, and diarrhea...' (IPCC 2014: 37).

Clearly, then, low-income countries will be most adversely affected in relation to health by climate change. 'Loss of healthy life years in low income African countries, for example, is predicted to be 500 times that in Europe' (McMichael et al. 2008: 3). Yet, the 'developed' world will by no means be immune, as the IPCC (2014: 37) points out: '[H]igher income populations may also be affected by extreme events, emerging risks, and the spread of impacts from more vulnerable populations.' More limited access to social resources among many in high-income countries will maximise exposure to effects such as those caused by Hurricane Katrina in New Orleans (United States) in 2005. Research into the social effects of this natural disaster found that African-Americans and others on low incomes, who were supposed to be protected by the levee system that collapsed, were the hardest hit (Hartman and Squires 2007). Institutional racism and class produced dramatically inequitable health results. In fact, the most devastating effects of natural disasters in the 20th and 21st centuries have been on those who generally experience the greatest adversity produced by class, gender and ethnicity (Donner and Rodriguez 2008). According to the IPCC (2014), the adverse health effects of climate change will be similarly socially patterned.

Physical threats to air, water and soil that pose major health challenges, particularly in relation to health equity, also demonstrate inadequate regulation. Air quality, for instance, is severely diminished by widespread pollutants that derive mainly from 'industrial processes, power production and personal transport' (Baum 2008: 320), making it predominantly an urban problem globally, especially in low and middle-income countries, such as India and China. Contaminated and degraded water affect 'developing nations' more than their affluent counterparts, particularly with respect to high mortality from waterborne diseases, such as diarrhoea, cholera, typhoid and dysentery. These arise predominantly from poor sanitation, as the WHO/UNICEF Joint Monitoring Programme for Water and Sanitation (WHO and UNICEF 2013) reported. By the end of 2011, an estimated 768 million people globally did not have access to piped water on premises or other kinds of water improvements (WHO and UNICEF 2013). More than 80 per cent of these people lived in rural areas, mainly in sub-Saharan Africa and Oceania. At the same time, 'there were 2.5 billion people who still did not use an improved sanitation facility. The number of people practising open defecation decreased to a little over 1 billion, but this still represents 15% of the global population' (WHO and UNICEF 2013: 5). Sub-Saharan Africa, Oceania and South Asia were most affected.

Certain industrial chemicals, such as PCBs (polychlorinated biphenyls), DDT and industrial waste products (dioxins, for example) are described as 'persistent organic pollutants', and are highly contaminating of water and soil. They are ubiquitous, permeating water and soil systems wherever industrialisation and industrialised products containing these chemicals have been used – from manufacturing to commercial and household operations of all kinds. They are understood to have severe but insidious and cumulative health effects, such as damage to endocrine and immune systems, various cancers, infertility among men and women, heart disease and genetic defects among males (Baum 2008). Though now banned in the United States, PCB production has left widespread 'legacy' pollution. This prevails in greater concentrations in industrial settings and nearby residential areas that are disproportionately populated by working class and ethnic minorities, exposing them to high risk of the health dangers associated with these chemicals.

Regulation and deregulation: Social division and politics

Regulation and deregulation, then, exert enormous effects on health disparities, both within and between countries. As the following section explains, these state processes operate hand-in-hand with re-distribution through taxation and transfers. Before moving on to discussing these, however, it is important to recognise that regulatory interventions, including their absence or abolition, are closely associated with intense social conflict arising from social division and inequality, and its expression in organised political activity. In relation to the latter, various interests usually form groups or establish associations to influence and direct the making and un-making of laws and rules involved in regulation. Associations of employers, large industry leaders, and health, medical and welfare service providers, trade unions, environmental protection bodies, women's rights groups, Indigenous peoples' councils and so on are common examples. They engage with political parties, government and opposition politicians, and senior decision makers and advisers in public-sector bureaucracies to press their claims for regulation or deregulation. In some cases, the beneficiaries of social division, such as large corporations and employers, are benefited by state regulatory actions, while in others it is those who more regularly bear the costs of inequality who can be advantaged. For example, the Australian Government recently announced major cuts to the funding and staffing of the Australian Securities and Investments Commission (ASIC), which regulates companies and their financial dealings, proposing that companies should be able to regulate themselves (Martin 2014). Such a development represents a significant withdrawal of government control of corporate activities and a green light for more laissez-faire market practices and increased profitability. At the same time, the New South Wales State Government has imposed increased restrictions on the sale of alcohol, especially in licensed premises that are part of the 'night-time economy'. Such regulation reduces the profitability of these businesses but reduces the risk of serious health-related harms associated with liberal access to alcohol (Loxley et al. 2005). Those at greatest risk of such damage have been young people, the majority of whom do not have access to accumulated social and economic resources upon which they might draw in the event of alcohol-related damage – both to themselves and others.

However, as the distribution of social resources and health disparities shows, while the democratic state in rich capitalist societies may address health inequity through regulatory interventions, it does not make policies and pass laws that challenge the foundations of capitalist accumulation. For example, there is no regulation anywhere on how much private property and wealth individuals may accumulate. This is not to say that all states are the same in terms of the extent to which they contribute to social inequality. The Nordic states, for example, have adopted approaches to rule and governance that have generated the least social and health disparity in the world (OECD 2013b). As the following outlines, the main mechanism they have used to achieve such an out-come is re-distribution through taxation and transfers.

Re-distribution through taxation and transfers

Taxation and other government imposts have been defining features of states since they first appeared, as explained previously in this chapter. In fact, states cannot exist without them because they provide the main financial means for their operations. From a sociological perspective, *taxation is a social practice that distinguishes the state from other domains of social process such as class and gender*. It plays a critical role in both the production and reduction of social in-equality and health inequity, but it does so in partnership with other practices of income and wealth re-distribution, sometimes called *tax transfers*. The most lucrative sources of state revenue in high-income countries are generally taxes on income and profits (paid as company tax) (OECD 2013d). In fact, these furnish most of the state's income, amounting to an average of 62 per cent of all government revenues in high-income countries (OECD 2013d). In all OECD countries and most others throughout the world, a *progressive* approach to in-come tax applies. This means that rates of taxation increase with the level of income earnt and declared by the citizenry. Income includes wages, salaries, interest on investments, dividends and so on. Such an approach is regarded as fairer than a flat or standard tax rate because those who earn more are regarded as being able to contribute more to the public purse as a proportion of their in-comes. Yet, in many high-income countries, those who earn more or own more (as wealth) pay little or no tax. In Australia, for example, 'only 2% of income earners pay the top rate of tax' (Hodgson 2014). Those identified as the very wealthiest individuals by the Australian Taxation Office – numbering 2600 in 2010 and each controlling AUD 30 million or more – 'contributed 1.2% of the tax paid by individuals and 5% paid no tax' (Hodgson 2014).

By contrast, indirect taxes such as the VAT (value-added tax) in Britain and the GST (goods and services tax) in Australia, and other consumption taxes on purchased goods or services (most notably property and excise taxes), are flat taxes and are recognised as imposing a progressively heavier financial bur-den on those with the lowest incomes. Yet, they are regarded by governments and their administrations as a more reliable and easier way for states to collect revenue because they are generally paid compulsorily at the point of purchase and virtually on most of what we buy. Constituting 32 per cent of high-income countries' government revenues on average (OECD 2013d), they are also regarded by some as better for economic growth than direct taxes (OECD 2011a), despite their exacerbation of social inequality.

Income tax payment is usually offset in most high-income countries with concessions, allowances and exemptions that operate as tax cuts. These favour income earnt as corporate profits over wages and salaries (Stilwell and Jordan 2007). This corporate advantage operates despite the fact that such tax concessions do not usually contribute towards economic growth and employment (Arnold et al. 2011). In some cases, especially in the Global South, tax breaks and other state financial incentives are paid at such a high rate to resource-extractive enterprises, such as those associated with coal, iron, gold and oil mining, that only local elites enjoy any significant economic benefits (Lisk, Besada and Martin 2013). Recent European research suggests that since the Global Financial Crisis of 2009, 'the tax change that shows the most promise in terms of both increased growth and economic recovery is the reduction of income taxes (including social security contributions) *of those on low incomes* [emphasis added]. This would stimulate demand, increase work incentives and reduce income inequality' (Arnold et al. 2011: F76).

Pensions and benefits in OECD countries are generally paid from government revenues obtained through direct taxation or social security contributions. Recipients usually include those who are not labour market participants, most notably, older (over 65 years of age) or retired citizens, unemployed people, chronically ill or disabled people, and parents involved in the full-time care of babies and infants, among others. Together with state provision of services such as universal education, health care and welfare, these provisions represent the main means of re-distributing wealth and income in high-income nation states at least. Yet, levels of taxation and re-distribution among high-income countries vary greatly, corresponding with significant differences in the degree of social inequality and health disparity. These are most marked between the collection of the Nordic states of Denmark, Norway, Sweden and Finland, and the United States. Basically, the Nordic states have the highest rates of taxation on wealth and income, and the most egalitarian re-distributive mechanisms in the world, including extensive provision of public employment, a generous welfare system and other public goods and services, particularly child care, education (from pre-school to university), and health care. The Nordic states have achieved the least social inequity in the world and among the very best global health outcomes for the overwhelming majority of their citizens (United Nations 2013).

The United States, by comparison with all other OECD countries, exhibits the lowest rate of taxation – both direct and indirect – and among the lowest rates of state provision of benefits and services, especially related to unemployment, child care and health care (OECD 2013d). The United States' rates of health disparity are among the worst of all OECD countries (see Chapter 8) despite the fact that it remains the world's biggest economy with the largest national share of the world's wealth (see Chapter 3).

Corporatisation and marketisation

A further means by which neo-liberal states have exercised rationalised governance, intensifying social inequality, is *corporatisation* (Shleifer and Vishny 1994). Basically this involves organising and managing the activities of public sector agencies or government departments according to the principles and practices governing private companies. Politicians and senior bureaucrats focus on cutting costs and maximising 'outputs', 'in line with a private sector approach rather than a traditional bureaucratic one' (Lewis 2005: 49). Rationalisation occurs through centralised control of senior management in planning, setting targets and monitoring performance. Allied to the operation of corporatisation is *marketisation*. According to Anneli Anttonen and Gabrielle Meagher (2013: 16), 'competition and customer choice are central in marketised service systems'. They say that marketisation also depends on the involvement of private actors or for-profit companies in the production and distribution of public services. Corporatisation and marketisation were pioneered in the regimes of the 1980s under the leadership of the then-British Prime Minister, Margaret Thatcher, and the then-United States President, Ronald Reagan. The combination of the two has been most pronounced in the United Kingdom, 'where the term, the "new public management" (or NPM) refers to . . . reforms that encompass markets, competition and consumer choice along with managerialist approaches based on private sector theories and practices' (Lewis 2005: 50). In the 21st century, the reach and influence of the NPM – or 'enterprise government' in the United States – have shown no signs of diminishment. In fact, they appear to be on the rise, even insinuating themselves among the Nordic states, as recent research on the marketisation of elder care there shows (Meagher and Szebehely 2013).

One of the hallmarks of corporatisation and market governance has been a radical transformation in determining the value of public sector production and distribution of goods and services, especially in health policy and health care. Consistent with an 'outputs' focus, identifying value in terms of efficiency based on narrow and quantifiable performance measures has become widespread. Patient 'throughput' is an especially common measure, indicated by the number of patients attended by practitioners, such as those in hospital accident and emergency departments, or the length of patients' stay in public hospitals (Hollingsworth 2008). Creating competition among different providers and terminating public-sector agencies' delivery of services in favour of private or 'not-for-profit' contractors and businesses has transformed the work of public-sector health care delivery irrevocably. 'For-profit' or commercial organisations have increased significantly, indicating the increased *privatisation* of health systems in Australia, Canada and the United Kingdom (Collyer and White 2011, Whiteside 2011, Pollock and Price 2011).

Corporatisation and marketisation have brought with them the growing *commodification* of health care – a development discussed in depth in Chapter 8. This has involved a profound change in 'the public' and how we understand it in relation to health care. After World War II in most Anglo democracies such as Australia, Canada, New Zealand and the United Kingdom, the idea of citizenship began to incorporate social as well as basic political rights. Education, housing, social welfare and health care came to be identified as social entitlements necessary for democratic participation (Dwyer 2010, O'Connor, Orloff and Shaver 1999). In the process, health care developed as a public good that was to be secured and distributed by states. The marketisation of health, by contrast, renders 'the public' an aggregation of individual *consumers* of health services, supposedly free to choose among different producers or distributors (Harley et al. 2011). As market players, citizens have no claims to goods and services as entitlements, and states no obligation to secure access to them. Such an approach has inequitable social consequences because, as previously explained, individual consumers are not all equal in terms of the resources they bring to negotiating market dynamics and purchasing commodities – including health care (Rylko-Bauer and Farmer 2002). Those with superior access to social resources, especially education and social networks, do better. Further, medical market providers are more likely to go where the money is most easily made, and costs, both financial and social, are minimised (White 2000). In health care this is usually in more affluent and resourced urban regions. As a result, outer-urban, rural and remote areas with concentrations of marginalised people tend to be poorly served and have equitable access to health care severely compromised (Palmer and Short 2014, Schofield

2012b). As Chapter 8 shows in detail, the corporatisation and marketisation of health care is one of the most significant contributors to health inequity, not only in the Global North but in the Global South as well.

Individualisation

The corporatisation and marketisation of public services with the advent of neo-liberal governance have been fortified by the process of *individualisation*. Some sociologists have proposed that individualisation is a distinctive feature of modernity (Beck 1992, Beck and Beck-Gernsheim 2002). It is identifiable primarily as a relationship in which people are emancipated from traditional social ties, bonds and commitments, allowing individuals to construct their own lives and make their own decisions. Individualisation has developed as a process of public governance through a combination of discourses and practices that establish individuals as being *responsible* for their own lives and not expecting governments and public sector agencies to support or subsidise them. Individualised governance in relation to health represents being poor, overweight or obese, with a gambling or other addiction, or even a chronic illness or disability, especially if associated with a work injury, as failures of individual responsibility (Ferge 1997). Individuals are supposed to be responsible for their own health, rejecting drug use and excessive alcohol intake, exercising regularly, eating nutritious food in modest quantities, using sunscreen, attending the doctor's surgery for check ups as they hit middle to older age, and taking out private health insurance cover (Harley et al. 2011).

Individualisation as a process of contemporary governance operates as though all citizens have liberal access to agentic resources (see Chapter 3) that enable them to be responsible for their individual fates. The process is particularly visible in state health promotion and harm-minimisation strategies that give emphasis to the role of information and education in health risks, assuming that individuals are completely free to choose a 'healthy lifestyle' (Cockerham 2005). Instead of focusing on the barriers to equality that underpin health inequities through well-resourced regulatory interventions, for instance, the state targets citizens' individually damaging behaviours, appealing to their rationality to control or stop them. For example, healthy eating campaigns warn people about the harms caused by the excessive intake of refined carbohydrates, especially cane sugar, and saturated fats in their diets. At the same time, though most high-income countries have a regulatory framework for protecting food 'safety and hygiene', food manufacturers and distributors are not obliged to ensure that their produce conforms to dietary guidelines that eliminate or minimise ingredients associated with overweight or obesity. In the face of what some call an epidemic of obesity, the absence of such regulation effectively individualises a major social and health problem that has the heaviest effects on those with the least resources (Devaux and Sassi 2013). For the state to consider the health of its citizens largely as the consequence of *individual choice* means to put in place policies that, instead of redressing social inequality and health inequity, perpetuate the dynamics that produce them.

Participation: Marginalisation and exclusion

As explained earlier in this chapter, one of the most significant ways in which the modern democratic state distinguishes itself from its historical predecessors is the opportunity it offers for all citizens to participate in their rule and governance, primarily through parliamentary representation and the electoral system. Participation is the means by which citizens contribute to the collective 'intelligence' of democratic governance and are able to *voice* their concerns, ideally having them placed on government agendas for action. Participation, as we saw in Chapter 3, is an agentic resource and, as such, critical to people's health because it is a means by which they can act on and influence their lives. Greater access to participation, particularly with respect to political institutions, goes hand-in-hand with better health outcomes, as the WHO and other global experts have recently affirmed (WHO 2010c, Ottersen et al. 2014).

The institutional processes of representative democracy are supposed to work as the main method for citizens' political participation. In addition to the right to vote, these include becoming a member of a political party and participating in its activities, engaging in political protest supported by freedom of assembly and speech, contacting politicians and signing petitions. There are further participatory opportunities in what are described as *community* participation. For example, government departments invite citizens to participate through public consultation about their proposals for various projects, especially those that are likely to provoke opposition, such as the construction of major roadworks or other infrastructure that impinge adversely on people's property and their health. A more bureaucratically integrated mode of community participation in public governance involves government advisory committees and boards of publicly funded agencies such as public hospitals and statutory authorities. These are often comprised of various participants from 'the community', depending on the issue about which the government seeks advice and those the government identifies as relevant representatives of the community. 'The community' is a politically contested term – meaning that its identity and membership are largely determined by those who have the power to do so (Everingham 2003). It is more accurate, then, in terms of political participation to talk of *communities of interest*.

The process of participation in public governance, virtually all over the world, however, is not socially inclusive. It is characterised by deep social divisions that arise from institutionalised processes of marginalisation and exclusion. Within countries these result in the greater presence (Phillips 1995) and voices of wealthier and more highly educated men from dominant ethnic backgrounds. Their working-class counterparts, especially if they are women and/or from ethnic minorities, are less likely to be among those involved in influential policy and decision making in state apparatus (Hardy-Fanta 2006, Weller and Nobbs 2010). As a result, they are also more likely to be excluded from the politically competitive process of determining whose claims for state intervention, through regulation for instance, and resource allocation are to be recognised and endorsed. This marginalisation and exclusion is evident in the under-representation in arenas of state influence of those who bear most of the costs generated by the dynamics of social division and inequality. This varies enormously on a global basis, as the United Nation's data on gender representation in parliaments, for example, illustrates (UN 2013) (see also Chapter 4). However, the aggregate pattern in the composition of parliaments and the senior ranks of state organisations throughout the world, including the judiciary, reflects an under-representation of women, ethnic minorities and Indigenous peoples, and an over-representation of men whose socio-economic status indicates greater class privilege (Connell 2009).

Despite the obvious inequalities in the representation of social constituencies, few democratic states have been successful in fixing the problem. Some of the Nordic states have established a quota system to ensure equal representation of men and women in their parliaments and on the boards of large companies (Borchorst and Siim 2008). In relation to voluntary associations, some governments have mandated equity provisions for those that want to be considered for public funding. For example, in Australia, public funding to support community based national sporting organisations has been conditional on the adoption of gender-equity principles in the election of their boards (Adriaanse and Schofield 2013). One of the most direct interventions in some states, particularly in Europe, to promote greater equity of participation in workplace management to improve health is through the compulsory establishment of workplace health and safety committees, including in the private sector. Membership of such committees usually requires a majority of employees who have considerable powers over work processes and conditions that pose risks to their health (Walters and Nichols 2007).

Conclusions

Though not often recognised as a social dynamic, the state plays a critical role in the making and un-making of social inequality and health inequity. Like its other major counterparts – class, gender, ethnicity and indigeneity – it is characterised by tangible features. Government offices and buildings, symbols such as national flags, state employees and public transport illustrate the materiality of the state. The state is also widely understood as 'a collection of institutions, including the parliament (government and opposition political parties), the public sector bureaucracy, the judiciary, the military, and the police' (Williams and Lawlis 2014: 444). However, while the state encompasses these features, from a sociological perspective that seeks to understand how the state works in relation to social inequality and health inequity, this chapter has emphasised the state as a specific arena of social process. Its distinctiveness stems from what lies at the heart of this process – governance and rule. This is what the institutions of the state do and why they exist. What animates the process are power and politics – or struggles and contests among conflicting interests for resources. There are two main types: symbolic resources – mainly rights and authorisations (to marry, to consume alcohol, to be a citizen, to work as a professional and to enter a workplace to conduct health and safety inspections, for example); and material resources (such as pensions and benefits, tax concessions and public infrastructure).

Central to what this chapter has proposed is that the state is characterised by the exercise of centralised authority. For much of its existence, this authority has operated autocratically and often despotically through monarchical or imperial rule. However, the contemporary state requires popular consent to legitimate its existence and operation. Force remains an integral feature of the modern state in order to enforce its rule, but the exercise of centralised authority also relies heavily on general acceptance of 'how we do things round here'. Political conflict and struggle continue but with representative democracy and rationalised governance they have become institutionalised in many parts of the world, through parliamentary and party politics, for instance. However, the interests that accompany such contestation are not simply many, diverse and random. Rather, there are structures of interest that express the tensions in social divisions such as class, gender, ethnicity and indigeneity. The ways in which such tensions get played out in state processes can reproduce or dissolve old relations of social inequality, re-forming and creating new ones.

With the rise of neo-liberalism in governance and rule since the 1980s, centralised authority has increasingly favoured the interests of markets and corporations, deepening global division and intensifying social inequalities. This development has been played out through a number of processes that are now central to how the contemporary state works, at least in the rich democracies of the world. Regulation and deregulation, re-distribution through taxes and transfers, corporatisation and marketisation, individualisation and marginalisation or exclusion from participation are foundational. Regulation, re-distribution and participation have prevailed as integral to the operation of states prior to neo-liberalisation, significantly reducing health inequities in the Global North. However, their re-making in the face of a vigorous commitment to neo-liberal governance poses enormous barriers globally to the advancement of health equity, as the following chapter illustrates in depth.

Questions for discussion

1   What do you understand by 'the state' from a sociological perspective?
2   When did states first emerge, and why? What were the defining features of early states?
3   What are nation states?
4   What is rationalised governance? When, where and why did it develop?
5   Why has the democratic state been described as a neutral umpire?
6   What does it mean to say that the state is partisan?
7   What is the relationship between the state and major social divisions such as class, gender, ethnicity and indigeneity?
8   What is neo-liberalism?
9   What are the main processes involved in neo-liberal governance and rule in most contemporary democracies in the Global North?
10   How do the processes of neo-liberal governance and rule advance health inequities? Who are most adversely affected?

8 Health care and health

Overview

Toni Schofield and Michelle Donelly

- What is the globally dominant form of health care organisation? How does it work?

- What is the most effective form of health care in terms of advancing the health of most of the world's peoples? How does it work?

- What are the major social dynamics responsible for the prevailing patterns of health care both within and between countries globally?

Iraq, 1950s

In the 1950s, archaeologists found a traumatised Neanderthal skeleton in northern Iraq in the Shanidar caves. Their examination of the remains showed that it was the skeleton of a man who had lived between 40 000 and 115 000 years ago and who had begun life with a stunted arm, a large part of it which he had lost some time later. It is likely that without the use of both arms the man had used his mouth for some tasks, such as scraping or cutting – because his teeth were very severely ground down. He had also lost two front teeth, probably in another accident. At some point in this life from thousands of millennia ago, something or somebody had delivered a sharp blow to the top of the man's head…This was accompanied by another, harder blow that had caused the left side of his face to be shattered, most probably destroying his sight on this side as well. Somehow, he had struggled on long enough to develop severe and crippling arthritis. '[A]round his fortieth birthday the roof over his cave hearth collapsed, ending his saga and his troubles.' (Wood: 1979: 22)

According to the author of the above account, 'Nandy', as the discoverers of the skeleton called him, revealed certain social circumstances of the time. 'The presence of enemies who perpetrated the skull damage' (Wood 1979: 23) is the most obvious; but even more telling is that Nandy could not have survived for as long as he did without receiving sustained nursing from his kin or clan. This fact underlines one of the key ideas developed in this chapter: that health care is a *social* phenomenon that is critical to human health. Health care, however, is not homogeneous. Human societies have been remarkably inventive over time and across the globe in organising how they attend to people when they are sick or injured, or living with a chronic condition or impairment, or giving birth or dying. Yet, in the 21st century, some kinds of health care are far more effective in enhancing peoples' health than others, as the evidence presented below shows. What is critical to the difference in efficacy and degree of health equity is how health care is socially organised, or how it works as a social process (Starfield, Shi and Macinko 2005).

Like all the social processes discussed in the previous chapters, power and politics are central. From a sociological perspective, there are several major forces involved in these in relation to health care. One is *global division* (see Chapters 3 and 6) and the dominance of *markets* and international *corporations*. These are especially influential in respect to pharmaceutical corporations, such as Pfizer and Roche, and biomedical technologies and equipment, such as those produced by Johnson & Johnson and Siemens. Another focus is activity by nation *states* (see Chapter 7), primarily in relation to health care policy, health insurance and public funding and also in relation to other key social institutions such as the economy and finance, and education. These forces all have major effects on health, as we have seen in previous chapters. Nation-state policies, particularly in relation to the Global South, however, are heavily influenced by international financial institutions (see Chapters 3 and 6), mainly the International Monetary Fund (IMF) and World Bank. The WHO also plays a significant role, largely with respect to research and policy advice. Health care professionals are also key players, especially medical practitioners and their professional associations in the world's richest countries. The *professionalisation* and *dominance* of medicine in the health care division of labour, as we explain further on in this chapter, is a powerful social dynamic, but its influence on health equity depends on its relationship to state and corporate involvement in health care.

The international research-based evidence is unequivocal. The best health care arrangements, in terms of the health of the over-riding majority of the planet's 7 billion peoples, are those that ensure local access for all, without fees for care, and with a focus on trained providers who can *work with* – not on – individuals and communities in delivering care (Starfield 2011, WHO 2008, Baum 2008). For most peoples everywhere, both in the Global North and South, provision of optimal health care relies on a combination of core competencies (WHO 2006). Sound technical expertise based on good clinical knowledge and practice is critical but ineffective in the absence of other core expertise, such as basic knowledge and understanding of the specific social and environmental circumstances in which individuals and communities live and work. Maximising the effectiveness of such competencies relates to a further skill: working as a member of a 'multidisciplinary team' of health workers (WHO 2006: 25). This is not to diminish the role of specific clinical competencies such as medicine. Higher rates of 'physician density' in health care systems, for example, are strongly associated with lower rates of infant mortality throughout the world (Muldoon et al. 2011). Yet, optimal health care delivery demands far more than specialist medical expertise. The following turns to contrasting examples of health care organisation, and their effects on health: between Costa Rica and Cuba in the Caribbean, on the one hand, and the United States, on the other. This comparison is indicative of how health care is a variable social process that can work in very different ways but with surprisingly similar health results, particularly in relation to life expectancy and infant mortality.

Primary health care and universal health coverage in the Caribbean: Costa Rica and Cuba

'Between 1970 and 1983, Costa Rica cut general mortality by 40 percent, and infant mortality was reduced by 70 percent. A long term commitment to nationwide (universal) coverage in health care and key basic social services contributed crucially to this pattern' (WHO 2010a: 9). These improvements occurred in the face of minimal rural health services provision – fewer than 20 per cent of people (Munoz and Scrimshaw, 1995). Primary health care and environmental health programs underpinned this achievement, including education, promoting community organisation, access to clean drinking water, faeces disposal, vaccination, nutrition and family planning (Saenz, 1985). 'The Rural Health Program (RHP) identified areas of greatest need and trained community health workers to visit homes in their respective areas in order to improve health practices, sanitation and vaccination of children' (WHO 2010a: 9). This program was emulated in a parallel program introduced to address the health needs of slum dwelling communities in Costa Rica, with similar success (Saenz 1985).

Today, Costa Rica has a total population of almost 5 million, most of whom exist on very low incomes compared with their high-income counterparts. Ten per cent of Costa Rica's gross domestic product (GDP) is spent on health, and per-capita total health expenditure per annum is $1243 (2011). Life expectancy at birth is 79 years – the same as that of the United States (WHO 2014b). The dramatic improvement in general infant mortality, from 68 per 1000 live births in 1970 to 8.6 per 1000 live births in 2011 in Costa Rica is one of the world's 'modern marvels' in terms of health progress. Costa Rica is ranked 80 out of 189 on the World Bank's list of countries by the size of its GDP – an amount similar to that of Tunisia and Lebanon (World Bank 2014f). Its GDP is 0.003 per cent that of the American economy, the largest in the world.

Cuba is another example of a country with limited national wealth but with a health profile comparable to some OECD countries. Ranked 66 of 189 nations according to the size of its GDP, Cuba's economy is not markedly greater than that of Costa Rica. Its population health profile and mortality levels have been favourable since before the 1950s (WHO 2010a). However, these have improved further since the Cuban revolution in 1959. Today, Cuba has a total population of just over 11 million, with levels of per-capita income and percentage of GDP spent on health similar to Costa Rica. In 1959 the country's infant mortality rate was 60 per 1000 live births and life expectancy was 65.1 years. By 2012, infant mortality had improved dramatically, with six children per 1000 live births dying before the age of five years (WHO 2014b). Overall life expectancy also increased to 79 years – the same as that for the United States (World Bank 2013).

By contrast with most of their high-income counterparts, Costa Rica and Cuba have implemented comprehensive *primary health care* for individuals that forms the backbone of their health care systems (see Table 8.1). Key elements of the two countries' approach to health care include a focus on public health and disease prevention, especially the development of urban sanitation and clean water supply. The Caribbean approach also focuses on localised and decentralised health care delivery to ensure equitable access, and community participation in health programs – especially health education (WHO 2010a). It is also important to note the focus of Cuba's primary health care system on delivering high-quality programs to *everyone*, including formerly marginalised groups. This is distinct from the development of 'targeted' or parallel programs for marginalised or 'disadvantaged populations', which risk losing quality without the influence of more privileged and demanding constituencies (Forde, Rasanathan and Krech 2012). These services are backed up by community based urban and rural health programs in which health workers enter people's homes to deliver services designed to improve living conditions, health practices and vaccination of children, especially among the poorest and most marginalised.

TABLE 8.1 *Characteristics of different models of health care*

	TRADITIONAL MEDICAL, CLINIC-BASED CARE	LARGE-SCALE DISEASE CONTROL PROGRAMS	PEOPLE-CENTRED PRIMARY CARE
Focus	Pathology and cure	Targeted diseases	Fundamental health needs
Relationship between health care provider and recipient	Duration of a consultation	Duration of program implementation; may be a single vaccination	Continuing personal relationship
Program of health delivered	Episodic, curative care	Program-defined disease control interventions	Comprehensive, continuous and person-centred care
Responsibility/ role of health care provider	Safe treatment and advice delivered during consultation	Achieving disease control targets in a designated population	Health (along the life cycle) of a community to which they belong
Responsibility/ role of health care recipients	Consumers or patients of the care they purchase	Population groups are targets of disease control interventions	Individuals and communities are partners in managing their own health

Source: Adapted from WHO 2008: 43.

According to the WHO (2008), primary health care encompasses a combination of features that departs markedly from other kinds of 'conventional' health care, such as medical care provided in clinics or out-patient departments of hospitals, or disease control programs, as outlined below. At the heart of the primary health care approach is 'people-centred' care.

Central to Costa Rican and Cuban health advancement has been a specific approach to governance and rule (see Chapter 7) in which state-funded health care and welfare are critical. This commitment stems from the idea that there are public goods – such as health, education, and clean air, water and soil – that are essential to collective well-being. Accordingly, these resources cannot be left to markets to provide. Both Costa Rica and Cuba have ensured access for all to health care through *universal health insurance* (explained below).

Universal coverage

The availability of health care to all people regardless of its cost is referred to as the universal coverage of health care. Universal coverage reduces the negative effect of health care as a source of health inequity when people have no access to health care for financial reasons or face impoverishment in order to meet health costs. The essence of financing arrangements for universal coverage is to ensure protection against the financial costs of ill-health for everyone through substantial tax funding and/or national mandatory contributory health insurance (Gilson et al. 2007). Such an approach strengthens risk sharing and is associated with better average life expectancy and more equitable child survival rates (Gilson et al. 2007). Systematic reviews of available evidence show that the absence of universal coverage and reliance on user-pays, fee-for-service health care arrangements in low and middle-income countries lead to falling utilisation levels (LaGarde and Palmer 2006; Palmer et al. 2004). They impose barriers to service use that have greatest effect on those with the least resources: impoverishing women and lower-income and socially marginalised groups (CSDH 2008). From the WHO's perspective, universal coverage is a necessary requirement for primary health care (CSDH 2008).

International financial institutions and the market

The biggest threat to the internationally recognised social welfare and health systems in Costa Rica and Cuba, according to the WHO, is the IMF and the World Bank. In the 1980s, the emergence of neo-liberalism (see Chapters 3 and 7) had a devastating effect on the economies of many Latin American countries (Connell and Dados 2014). Costa Rica was one of them (Holden and Villars 2013). War broke out between the American-supported Contras, who operated out of Costa Rica, and the Nicaraguan government. Costa Rica was invaded by Nicaragua and then faced a huge influx of approximately 50 000 Nicaraguan immigrants by 1983 (International Organization for Migration 2014, Vargas 2005). Income from tourism and food exports to the United States dwindled, and Costa Rica was forced to establish an army, the first since its abolition in 1948. In order to survive the possible collapse associated with these developments, Costa Rica borrowed from the IMF, World Bank and USAID, but was consequently unable to meet the rising interest rates of deregulated financial markets. The terms of these loan arrangements stipulated that governments must introduce 'austerity measures', also known as Structural Adjustment Policies (SAPs). Typical measures included a reduction in government control of business and finance, the privatisation of public sector assets, reduction in social services and the promotion of foreign investment through trade and tax concessions. They operated according to principles based on, and advantageous to, the market economies and corporations of the global metropole (Lehndorff 2012, Robinson 2012).

Such measures have tended to cause unacceptable suffering, particularly to the poor and marginalised (Stiglitz 2002). In some countries, such as Greece, there has been widespread public hostility to such austerity measures, proposed in response to the effects of the Global Financial Crisis on the Greek economy. Greek resistance was fuelled by the threat of cuts to public expenditure and its effects, especially on health care and social welfare (Kondilis et al. 2013, Ottersen et al. 2014). Costa Rica and Cuba share this opposition, which has resulted in strained relations with the World Bank and the IMF. Though the countries differ in their arrangements for rule and governance – Costa Rica has an elected administration and Cuba's is centrally controlled and unelected – they nevertheless share similar approaches to economic management, foreign investment and 'the public good'. Both have implemented tight government controls over business and finance, and foreign investment, and have maintained strong provision for universal education, health care and welfare. Cuba's centralised decision making has contributed to better overall integration and cost-containment of health services. It has also enabled control over the country's finances and foreign investment, and independence from the financial institutions of the global metropole, affording protection of Cuba's health care organisation. Nevertheless, such independence has exposed the country to major economic and political challenges. In almost every industry, production has been declining (Mesa-Lago 2007). Public infrastructure is crumbling, and levels of unpaid public debt remain high, restricting access to international finance. At present this is mainly provided by countries with which Cuba has 'friendly relations', such as China, Venezuela, Russia and Brazil (Luis 2013). Resistance by Cuba's socialist leadership to engaging with its people to redress economic problems, however, poses a formidable barrier to Cuba's continuing advancement in health (Mesa-Lago 2007).

The World Bank and the IMF remain explicitly opposed to Costa Rica's and Cuba's approaches to governance, particularly their health care organisation and funding arrangements (People's Health Movement et al. 2011). The central issue of contention for these global financial institutions is the absence of a 'purchaser–provider split' (PPS) (Ottersen et al. 2014). This is a health care arrangement in which patients or clients must be able to obtain their health care from practitioners 'of their own choice'. Practitioners must be free to offer their services directly to those who seek them out. Public authorities are only permitted to participate in this arrangement as providers of contracts specifying the nature of the relationship between purchasers and providers (Tynkkynen, Keskimäki and Lehto 2013, Siverbo 2004). One of the main aims of the PPS is to create competition between providers because this is believed to prevent increased costs, improve greater efficiency, promote organisational flexibility, achieve better quality and enhance responsiveness of services to patient needs (Tynkkynen, Keskimäki and Lehto 2013). The PPS is a market-based mechanism for distributing health care (see Chapter 7). Since its introduction, however, there is no strong evidence that it has made any significant difference in terms of the outcomes it was supposed to produce (Tynkkynen, Keskimäki and Lehto 2013, Siverbo 2004).

The insistence by the World Bank and IMF that the most effective and efficient way to organise health care is through the application of market-based principles amounts to an endorsement of higher private expenditure by individuals on health care. The WHO's Commission on the Social Determinants of Health (2008) states that there is no evidence to support this approach in terms of improving health outcomes or systems efficiency, especially in low-income countries, as the following extract outlines:

> Higher private sector spending [relative to all health expenditure] is associated with worse health-adjusted life expectancy, while higher public and social insurance spending on health [relative to GDP] is associated with better health-adjusted life expectancy (Mackintosh and Koivusalo 2005). Moreover, public spending on health is significantly more strongly associated with lower under-5 mortality levels among the poor (Houweling et al. 2005). The Commission for the Social Determinants of Health considers health care a common good, not a market commodity. Underlying these reforms is a shift from commitment to universal coverage to an emphasis on the individual management of risk. Rather than acting protectively, health care under such reforms can actively exclude and impoverish. (p. 95)

The United States, biomedicine and private or corporatised health care

The United States is geographically located in close proximity to Cuba and Costa Rica but shares little in common with its Caribbean neighbours in relation to social organisation and governance, including health care arrangements. The United States is described as a *liberal democracy* in which the relationship between the state and individual freedom is fundamental. Basically, in a liberal democracy, the public good is understood in terms of the protection of individual rights, particularly in relation to private property, freedom of speech, assembly and religion. Citizens obey the state to the extent that the state protects these rights, enshrined in the Constitution of the United States. Accordingly, the state has no business in protecting *collectivities*, except insofar as this is necessary to protect individual rights such as those of religious minorities, and the 'national interest'. Liberal democracies favour and support market-based economic activity because it is viewed as best able to maximise individuals' needs at the same time as it ensures the growth of private property.

The United States, of course, is also a much more populous country than its Caribbean neighbours, with a total population of 318 million (2012) and a much greater proportion of its GDP spent on health care. In fact, 18 per cent of GDP is allocated to overall health care expenditure – the highest in the world – with per-capita health expenditure 20 times greater than that of Cuba. American life expectancy and child mortality rates, however, are virtually the same as Cuba's, as previously mentioned (WHO 2014b) (see Figure 8.1).

Though Figure 8.1 indicates that American life expectancy is slightly higher than that of Cubans', more current data show that the rates between Cuba and the United States are the same, as previously indicated. The average rates of life expectancy and child mortality in the United States, by contrast with both Cuba and Costa Rica, actually mask deep health disparities within the population. For example, in the American state of Mississippi, infant mortality is equivalent to that of Costa Rica, at 10 deaths per 1000 live births, but in Minnesota it is 6 per 1000 live births (United Health Foundation, UNHF 2011). By contrast with Costa Rica's universal health coverage, 19 per cent of people in Mississippi have no health insurance, while 9 percent have no coverage in Minnesota (UNHF 2011). As Chapter 3 outlined, there are major disparities in life expectancy across the United States by income, education and other socio-economic indicators. Ethnicity and racism have similar effects, as Chapter 5 showed. There is a life expectancy difference of 15 years for men and 13 years for women between African-Americans and White Americans (Murray et al. 2006). International comparisons indicate that in the United States, life expectancies in some counties are 50 years behind those of the best-performing nations, while other American counties do better than the best-performing nations. This geographic variation in life expectancy is more pronounced in the United States than in the United Kingdom, Canada or Japan. Recent evidence (Kulkarni et al. 2011) indicates that between 2000 and 2007 health disparities deteriorated further despite per capita health expenditure being higher in the United States than any other nation in the world.

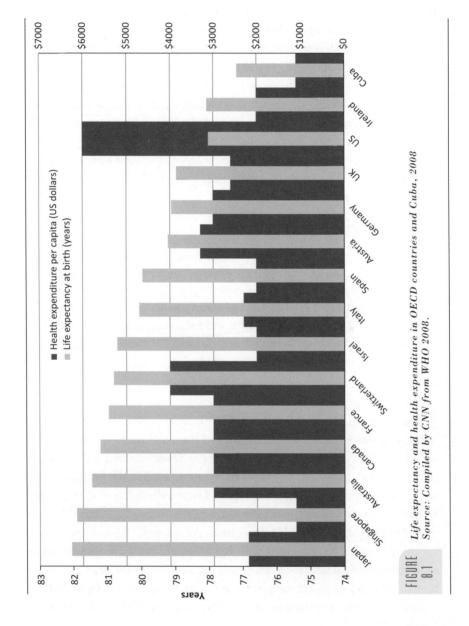

FIGURE 8.1 *Life expectancy and health expenditure in OECD countries and Cuba, 2008*
Source: Compiled by CNN from WHO 2008.

In contrast to both Costa Rica and Cuba, health care in the United States is dominated by a *biomedical* approach, which takes a focus on disease and high-tech medicine to *cure* it. It is a market-based system with *user-pays, fee-for-service* health care delivery. Patients purchase medical and hospital services directly from providers without government intervention. There is no primary health care along the lines proposed by the WHO, and no universal health coverage. Not surprisingly, then, access to health care depends mainly on market-based health coverage, or private health insurance whereby people have individual responsibility for buying coverage by paying premiums to a health insurance company. Market-based health insurance basically means that access to health care for the majority of Americans depends on their ability to pay for health insurance. The United States Census Bureau (DeNavas-Walt, Proctor and Smith 2011) reported that 64 per cent of the population was covered by private health insurance in 2010, and 31 per cent by government health insurance:

> The U.S. Census Bureau broadly classifies health insurance coverage as private coverage or government coverage. Private health insurance is a plan provided through an employer or a union or purchased by an individual from a private company. Government health insurance includes such federal programs as Medicare, Medicaid, and military health care; the Children's Health Insurance Program (CHIP); and individual state health plans. (DeNavas-Walt, Proctor and Smith 2011: 25)

Insurance cover through Medicare or Medicaid involves complex application and eligibility arrangements, and long delays in achieving registration, which poses significant barriers for people who often have no backup from family or friends, and with low levels of education and literacy. According to the United States Department of Health and Human Services (2011), children and older adults are significantly more likely to be uninsured if they are living in poverty and, therefore, also more likely not to receive the health services and medication they need because of cost. Those with least access to material resources pay the highest price in terms of health damage that could be prevented or mitigated with early intervention. For example, African-Americans are more likely to be diagnosed with late-stage breast cancer and colorectal cancer than their fellow citizens. People with low incomes have less access to diabetic services and consequently are more likely to experience diabetic complications and hospital admissions (Agency for Health Care Research and Quality 2012).

The costs of market-based health care in the United States are among the highest in the world. Of all bankruptcy filings in 2007 in the United States,

62 per cent were partly the result of medical expenses. Yet, medical insurance appears to have provided no guarantees against financial ruin, with 75 per cent of those declared bankrupt having actually paid up their health insurance subscriptions (Himmelstein et al. 2009). The high cost of health care is associated with a number of factors. Employment-based medical insurance and out-of-pocket payments have increased well beyond other consumer price rises (Gilson et al. 2007). Unnecessary interventions and over-servicing by medical providers are endemic; and with 'top-of-the-line' insurance cover taken out by a large proportion of the population, many expect, and are able to pay for, hi-tech, specialist medical treatment even when 'medical indications' do not warrant it (Farrell et al. 2008). Rates of pharmaceutical prescription and medical imaging procedures are higher than any other OECD country (UNHF 2011). Yet, the factors associated with inflated health care costs themselves need to be explained – a task addressed later in this chapter.

In recent times under the Obama Government, in order to increase access to health care in the United States, reforms have been introduced with the Affordable Health Care Act. However, they have met with robust opposition. The opposition Republican Party has argued that the reforms are not consistent with the free-market principles or market-driven approaches they *believe* regulate the costs of health insurance, despite the overwhelming evidence that this is not the case (Roy 2014). The American Medical Association supports the wider provision of health insurance under the Affordable Health Care Act but opposes quality outcomes reporting, and is concerned about the regulation of pricing for medical services, including payments to physicians (Medicare News Group 2014). Pharmaceutical companies have supported the increase in rebate payments on drug costs to older adults and people with disabilities. Yet, they oppose mandatory reporting of the direct and indirect payments they make to physicians and teaching hospitals to encourage prescription of their drugs (Brownlee 2012, Campbell et al. 2010).

The social relations of Costa Rican, Cuban and American health care approaches

It is evident, then, that access to primary health care – including universal health coverage – positively influences health by reducing the incidence, suffering and costs of communicable and non-communicable diseases (Lopez et al. 2006, Beaglehole et al. 2008). It is also critical to the prevention of maternal mortality, newborn deaths and postnatal deaths, and of mortality of children under 5 years of age (Bhutta et al. 2008, Rohde et al. 2008), not only outside high-income countries but within them as well (Muldoon et al. 2011). Primary health care is the most advantageous approach to health because of the way in which it operates as a social and embodied process. Most diseases, both communicable and non-communicable, and complications of pregnancy and childbirth, are embodied conditions that respond best to treatments and services provided before onset (such as vaccination), at early onset or over the course of their duration. Through such provision, these embodied conditions can be prevented or cured, or the suffering and discomfort associated with them mitigated. This means that access to care is critical. The most accessible care is that made freely available and located within areas in which people live and work, namely, primary health care. Competent providers who are people-centred and who work together towards advancement of their community's health are crucial, as previously mentioned. The social relations of primary health care, then, are characterised by a focus on local communities or groups of people in residential areas or workplaces, and the provision, at no cost, of clinical and social expertise in these locations to promote people's health, usually at health centres or regular mobile clinics. Such an approach reflects what some sociologists describe as social relations of *solidarity* and *cooperation* (Crow 2002). There are further significant dimensions, as illustrated above, particularly community health programs and what is called 'intersectoral collaboration'. This involves public-sector agencies working actively with health service providers to prevent obvious sources of disease and injury, such as the lack of sanitation or clean drinking water, or the production of toxic substances in soil, air and waterways, or damaging employment and workplace equipment. Sanitation and clean drinking water were recently identified by a study based on 136 United Nations member countries as one of two main 'factors' necessary for health care systems to achieve low rates of maternal, child and infant mortality (Muldoon et al. 2011).

This model of primary health care has no connection with markets or profit-making, as illustrated in the countries of Costa Rica and Cuba. Clinical visits, basic medications, community programs and so on are not sold by service providers to clients or patients. The social relations of biomedicine and private health care in the United States, by contrast, are based on market dynamics. Biomedicine focuses on the individual, in particular on organic function, and the development and application of a range of technical treatments – including surgical, chemical, radiation, laser, stem-cell and tissue transfer (blood, organs and embryos, for example) – to address and cure organic dysfunction (Waldby and Mitchell 2006, Clarke and Shim 2011). The social relations of market-based care are characterised by the buying and selling of health services – on a user-pays or fee-for-service basis – and medical products made by corporations to make profits. As disclosed by its operation in the United States, access depends on market dynamics, with clients having to pay directly out of their own pockets or by buying individual health insurance (OECD 2013c). Competition among biomedical service and product providers is believed to offer the best health care and treatments, and health insurance companies do likewise to provide the best health coverage or service access at the most competitive prices. It is expected that an individual's health will be optimised by this competitive process, the high-tech expertise of medical practitioners and the medical code of ethics by which practitioners are bound to protect and promote individual patient health. The highly individualistic character of the social relations of market-based care renders any kind of social solidarity related to health and health care superfluous.

Health care in the Gobal North: Medical markets, publicly subsidised

Health care expenditure involves approximately 10 per cent of the world's GDP. Most of this expenditure occurs in the high-income countries of the Global North and its affiliates in places like Australia and New Zealand. Health care in these countries is largely shaped by market-based biomedicine but governments play a significant role. For example, in 2011 in the 30 OECD countries, the average *public* or government share of *all* health expenditure on medical services was 78 per cent and 54 per cent on medical goods (including pharmaceuticals) (OECD 2013c). Only six countries had lower rates for both, including Australia (73 and 45 per cent, respectively) and the United States (50 and 32 per cent, respectively). However, in most OECD health care contexts, there is a mix of private and government ownership of health care. In 2013, among 14 OECD countries, including all of the Anglo-democracies, 'primary care' (or care by a local general medical practitioner, or GP) was predominantly privately owned in all except for Sweden (Thomson et al. 2013). In these same countries, hospital provision revealed a different pattern, with most either publicly owned, as in England, New Zealand, Denmark, Sweden, Norway, Italy and Switzerland, or dominated by a combination of public and private (not-for-profit) as in Australia, Canada, France, Germany, Japan and the United States. The Netherlands was the only country without public hospital provision (Thomson et al. 2013). Private (for-profit) hospital provision occurred in virtually all countries but at negligible levels in Japan and the Scandinavian countries, and at the highest levels in the United States, Germany and Australia. In Australia, for example, 68 per cent of all hospital beds and three out of every five hospitalisations were in public hospitals (AIHW 2013a). Private hospitals operated as both for-profit and not-for-profit.

The majority of hospitals in high-income countries, then, as exemplified by the 14 OECD members described above, do not operate in order to make profits. Most are sites of sophisticated biomedical service delivery, characterised by routine use of complex medical procedures, pharmaceuticals, medical goods and high-tech medical equipment. Supplies needed by hospital medical services derive from markets. The sellers, predominantly large corporations that specialise in producing pharmaceuticals, biotechnological and high-tech medical equipment, as previously mentioned, are located in the global metropole. The use of pharmaceutical products, of course, is not confined to hospitals. Prescriptions by 'primary care' providers, mainly GPs, account for the large proportion of the market, especially antibiotics, antihypertensives, cholesterol-lowering drugs, antidiabetics and antidepressants (OECD 2013c). These comprise the main biomedical technologies used by primary care doctors in high-income countries to treat illness and disease.

The 'top 10' pharmaceutical corporations, ranked by revenue, are based in the United States, the United Kingdom, France and Switzerland (Forbes 2013). In 2012, the combined sales revenue of the top 50, the largest of which also included Japanese and German corporations, amounted to more than 1000 billion dollars per year (Forbes 2013). At the same time, total biotechnological sales revenue among the top 50 corporations, again based almost exclusively in the Global North, reached over 600 billion dollars. When added together, revenues from pharmaceutical and biotechnology sales equated to approximately the size of the total GDP of India or Canada, ranked 10 and 11 respectively on the World Bank's list of economies by size of GDP (World Bank 2014f). These sales revenues exclude innumerable other products used in medical service provision, especially in hospitals, such as the devices and instruments used in the plethora of treatments now administered by biomedicine. For example, the top 40 manufacturers of medical devices in 2013 made almost 300 billion dollars in revenue (Forbes 2013). Private health insurance, like pharmaceutical, biotechnology and medical device manufacturing, is also mega-business. In the United States alone in 2012, health insurance companies raised over 1000 billion dollars in premiums (Martin et al. 2014).

While governments in most OECD countries fund most of the services provided by medical practitioners, they do not necessarily do so by employing them on a salaried basis, as they do with most other health care staff such as nurses. Most medical care is provided by GPs, though specialist medical care increasingly rivals the proportion of medical service provision by GPs (OECD 2013c). The majority of GPs in most OECD countries are self-employed or in private group practices (OECD 2013d, Thomson et al. 2013). In Australia, for instance, in 2012, approximately 85 per cent of general practice was undertaken mainly in the private sector (AIHW 2014). In most of the 14 OECD countries mentioned above, self-employed or private GPs charged a fee-for-service. This fee is not generally government regulated. However, a *capitation fee* – or a set amount per patient per year regardless of the number of patient visits, paid by a private or government insurance agency – is increasingly used in addition to fee-for-service by GPs in OECD countries such as England, Denmark, France, Italy, Sweden, the Netherlands and New Zealand (Thomson et al. 2013).

There is a division of labour in medical service provision in most high-income countries, with specialist and trainee medical practitioners performing most hospital-based work. Specialist doctors work in hospitals on both a salaried and fee-for-service basis in most OECD countries (OECD 2013d). It is evident, however, that many who are employed or salaried also operate their own fee-for-service practices outside public or not-for-profit hospitals, as happens commonly in Australia, the United Kingdom, the United States and Germany (Humphrey 2004: 163, Thomson et al. 2013). A significant proportion of income earnt by specialist medical practitioners in high-income countries is generated through market arrangements, even though much of their work takes place in public or not-for-profit settings. Not surprisingly, both specialist and general practitioners in all OECD countries earn rates of income that are markedly higher than the average wage, but specialists earn much more than their generalist counterparts (OECD 2013d).

Government expenditure on medical services usually takes the form of subsidies to the medical service industry. These subsidies are financed by government taxation usually earmarked as public health insurance schemes, such as Medicare in Australia. These reimburse medical fees for services, either directly to the doctor, such as 'bulk-billing' in Australia (Healy and Dugdale 2013), or through rebates to clients. In most OECD countries in which public health insurance schemes operate, clients also usually have to make *co-payments* (OECD 2013c), with the degree of *out-of-pocket expenses* varying. In France, for example, co-payments amount to 30 per cent of all medical service fees (OECD 2013c, Thomson et al. 2013) for which citizens can take out private health insurance to cover the cost. Unlike Medicare in the United States, Medicare in Australia is a universal health insurance scheme that means all Australian citizens have access to primary GP and hospital care regardless of income. Recent national health policy developments in Australia, however, are foreshadowing the introduction of co-payments that will terminate the 'universality' of health care access.Pharmaceuticals and other goods prescribed by medical practitioners in most OECD countries also usually need to be obtained through the market. Clients buy prescribed medical goods at pharmacies, but governments subsidise these purchases through arrangements such as the Pharmaceutical Benefits Scheme in Australia (Healy and Dugdale 2013). This form of government subsidy makes medical goods, especially medications, more affordable and accessible but clients must normally pay a proportion of the price themselves – a *co-payment* (OECD 2013c).

Clearly, medical practitioners in high-income countries occupy a central and powerful position in the organisation of health care. Much of their power derives from their independence from government control and the sale of their services through various biomedical markets. These include the market in primary care and its provision by GPs, and a wide range of specialist markets offering many different kinds of treatments. The capital and equipment that specialist practitioners need to produce their services are paid for by hospitals. Doctors do not incur such costs unless they have a share in the ownership of the hospital. In most high-income countries medical doctors also set their own fees, with very limited government regulation. The main role of governments in market-based medical care is that of public subsidiser. It does so in two ways: one, by rebating fees-for-service and, two, by funding public hospitals (including equipment and staff) to enable medical specialists to provide (or sell) their services without having to pay for the overheads involved. By any measure and by comparison with all other health care practitioners, the autonomy and power of biomedicine positions it as the dominant force in the organisation of global metropolitan health care (Allsop 2006: 449,

Willis 2006: 428). The historical foundations of medical dominance are complex (Starr 1982, Willis 1983, Larkin 1983, Coburn, Torrance and Kaufert 1983). From a sociological perspective, however, the process of *professionalisation* has been central in the rise of medicine and its continuing power in health care, as the following explains.

Professionalisation and medical sovereignty

Professionalisation is associated with the division of labour, mainly in the production of services. As previously discussed in Chapter 3, the division of labour has become characterised by a distinction that is virtually universal: between a minority that performs paid work involving the exercise of control and autonomy, and the majority who are employed to do what they are told to do – how, when, where and why. This distinction is one of the foundations of class and the hierarchies of power and authority that characterise it. One of the justifications for this hierarchy is that the controllers have *specialist knowledge* and *competence* required to keep work processes going and operating efficiently. Their possession of such know-how is indicated by the acquisition of relevant qualifications, usually conferred by universities.

Some sociologists suggest that the possession of specialist knowledge and expertise, and the credentials to prove it, constitute the basis for the differentiation between *professions* and *occupations*, and the differentials in remuneration, social recognition and power that accompany it (MacDonald 1995). There are other features as well, particularly a *code of ethics* that governs their work practices and commits them to the service of others, and a *licence* to practise their profession to the exclusion of all others, usually authorised by state agencies. Professions are identifiable, in other words, by characteristics or *traits* that distinguish them from other, 'mere' occupations. Prominent examples of professions recognised in this way are medicine, law, architecture, accountancy, dentistry, engineering, veterinary practice and so on.

Other sociologists argue that 'trait theory', with its focus on static categories or characteristics, cannot account for how some occupational groups have been able to secure the autonomy and control over work that characterises professions (Johnson 1995). Nor does it explain why some professionals within the same field, such as medical practitioners in health care, exercise far more power than others. While there are many occupations employed in health care, including complementary and alternative (CAM) health practitioners, only medical practitioners have the power to identify and certify what embodied conditions count as illness, disease, injury and impairment, and who can be socially recognised as sick or impaired. Further, other health professionals, such as nurses, while also disclosing similar traits to those of medicine, do not exercise anywhere near the degree of power and influence over health care and prevailing representations of health.

Clearly, medicine's control over its work is central to its power (Freidson 1970, Willis 1989), but it is the process of professionalisation and how it operates at the intersection of class, gender and state dynamics that explains how medicine succeeded in securing such control. Professionalisation is a combination of practices by which some groups within the division of labour take action to occupy a position of control and autonomy over their work and that of others, excluding competitors through the process. It is thus an inherently political process in which class dynamics are of central importance insofar as the collective financial and social advancement of an occupational group depends on demonstrating its superiority to other groups within a specific division of labour. As in the case of medicine, it can also depend on *excluding* or *subordinating* other occupational groups in the field of work involved (Willis 1983). Occupational superiority is usually associated with specialist knowledge gained through higher education – largely the preserve of those from middle and upper-class backgrounds. As the history of medicine's rise to pre-eminence in health care has shown, university education has been critical (Starr 1982, Willis 1983, Larkin 1983, Coburn, Torrance and Kaufert 1983). This is despite the fact that such education and training did not enable medical graduates to produce health outcomes that were any better than those of their competitors until around 1935 when sulphonamides, or early antibiotics, were introduced (Russell and Schofield 1986, McKinlay and McKinlay 2009). This new chemical treatment was most effective in reducing maternal mortality, much of which was associated with infection spread by poor medical hygiene. Some medical epidemiologists provide persuasive evidence that medical measures had very little to do with the decline in mortality that occurred after 1900 in wealthy countries, such as the United Kingdom and the United States (McKeown, Record and Turner 1975, McKinlay and McKinlay 2009).

Yet, class power, as we saw in Chapter 3, is often built on its interactions with the state. Not surprisingly, then, state dynamics are also integral to the power of the professions since an occupation that seeks to professionalise must demonstrate its superiority to a public authority responsible for licensing professions. Only the state can legitimate the claims of occupational groups to perform particular kinds of work to the exclusion of all others as part of its *regulatory* operations (see Chapter 7). Those who seek to professionalise their occupation and their work, such as medical practitioners, must engage in political organisation, lobbying governments to have their claims authorised as exclusive service providers. Such legitimation usually involves the state's endorsement of claims by professionalising groups attesting to their superiority – what some have called *legitimating discourse* (Sanders and Harrison 2008). State legitimation consolidates the boundaries that mark out professional service provision as exclusive territory. Only those with the designated specialist qualifications and expertise legitimated by a public authority are then permitted entry to practise in it. At the heart of medicine's professionalisation were its claims that only its specialist knowledge and practice could deliver genuine health benefits. Medicine's proponents argued that, by contrast with its competitors – such as homeopaths, midwives, herbalists, acupuncturists and so on – medicine was based on the rigours of 'scientific method' (Russell and Schofield 1986). Medicine's legitimating discourse enabled its practitioners to represent themselves and their practices to state agencies as superior to their competitors in order to secure their occupational advantage and class privilege. Such discourses continue to prevail in order to maintain medicine's position as the leaders in health care, but these discourses are not immutable. They can adapt to and even shape *policy* discourses to enable medicine to expand into new fields such as its entry into aged care after World War II and the development of geriatric medicine (Pickard 2010).

No less crucial in medicine's professionalisation, particularly with respect to strategies of exclusion and subordination, have been gender dynamics. Women were not explicitly excluded from practising medicine when legislation such as the British *Medical Act of 1858* was passed and 'established the first clear boundaries to the field of medicine and spelt out what its entry qualifications would be' (Pringle 1998: 24). However, because they were not permitted entry to university medical schools, women were not legally entitled to practise medicine. This sexual reproductive distinction (see Chapter 4) in admission requirements prevailed in all British colonies and the United States. Though it was formally removed by the turn of the 20th century, it was almost 100 years later before sex difference no longer operated in advantaging men over women in entering medical schools in countries such as Australia, the United Kingdom and the United States, when gender parity finally prevailed. By the late 19th century, medicine also began to colonise an arena of health care historically dominated by women – that of childbirth and the practice of midwifery. Almost 150 years later, midwives comprise the majority of the workforce in maternity care, but male-dominated specialist obstetrics dominate its organisation and practice in most high-income countries. Obstetricians occupy centre-stage in public policy that defines and prescribes appropriate maternity care, not necessarily with beneficial consequences for quality care (Reiger 2011).

At the same time, though numerically dominated by university educated women in most parts of the high-income world, nursing continues as a subaltern profession to medicine. This pattern is not 'all of a piece', as Deidre Wicks' (1998) Australian study of nurses and doctors at work reveals in closely observed detail. The boundaries between medicine and nursing in some health care settings, such as maternity wards, are more porous than a binary and category-based understanding of power dynamics would suggest (see Chapter 4). Senior nurses or midwives in such contexts, for example, often exercise more power and authority than trainee doctors. Yet, the *aggregate* picture in health care organisation remains one of medicine's dominance and nursing's subordination. As Evan Willis (1989) has explained, this dominance is in large part attributable to medicine's *sovereignty* beyond health care settings, in relation to prevailing societal understandings of health and illness, for instance. Allied health professions such as occupational therapy, social work, speech therapy, physiotherapy, orthoptics, podiatry, health information management and psychology are similarly positioned. Comprising around 10 per cent of the health workforce in Australia, the vast majority of these practitioners are women (Schofield 2009). However, in countries such as Australia and the United States, with opportunities for direct market-based service provision and fee-for-service delivery, some of these practitioners, such as physiotherapists and psychologists, have far more autonomy and control over their work than other allied health workers.

The dominant model of health care in the Global North and among its affiliates in the Global South, then, is organised largely through medical goods and services markets that are, in most cases, heavily subsidised by governments and some non-profit organisations, such as religious bodies. Service users or citizens pay for such services, through out-of-pocket expenditure, private health insurance premiums, government taxes or various combinations of these. Medical service providers, especially specialist practitioners, are major beneficiaries in terms of remuneration and control over health care organisation. Yet, large corporations that produce pharmaceuticals, substances, devices and so on for hospitals and primary care, and that sell private health insurance, derive the greatest financial dividends. What have been the health effects of this approach to health care organisation?

Health effects of biomedicine in the rich world

There is no doubt that modern biomedicine can deliver remarkable individual health benefits, especially in relation to conditions that can be cured through chemical or surgical interventions, and in easing pain, discomfort and suffering. There are many examples: hip and knee replacement operations, cure of bacterial infections and diseases, restoration of sight through surgery, repair of and survival from serious burns, wounds and fractures, and so on. Yet, there are also significantly major costs, apart from the obvious financial imposts.

One is the increasing number of frail and chronically ill older people whose survival is largely attributable to biomedical interventions – heart and vascular surgery, for example – but whose *quality of life* is extremely limited. The rise in longevity achieved in OECD countries primarily through social interventions, including public health, has not necessarily been accompanied by universal healthy old age (Blane 2006, Kendig and Browning 2010). This is not to say that the majority of older people – those over 65 years of age – are likely to have health conditions that render them chronically ill, frail and dependent on intensive care (AIHW 2012, Kendig 2004, Centers for Disease Control and Prevention 2007). Yet, the social divisions that render access to health unequal over the life course accumulate in older age, producing a substantial minority of older people who *are* chronically ill, frail and dependent on intensive care across high-income countries (OECD 2011b). The prevailing form of health care in the global metropole, however, is not oriented towards such care, making access to it constrained and linked to other social resources, especially wealth and income (OECD 2011b).

A further serious cost related to the former, then, is the restriction on access to health and support services for chronic illness, non-communicable diseases and seriously limiting – or disabling – conditions (Meekosha 2011). This cost is inextricably linked to the dominance of biomedicine. Health care in rich countries, and the money to finance it, centres on curative biomedicine – not chronic illness and disability that cannot be cured, at least not now or in the foreseeable future. Certainly, some pharmaceuticals and medical goods mitigate some of the physical and emotional distress associated with these conditions but ultimately it is a very different kind of care that is required – one that addresses the person, the physical and social environment in which he or she lives and works, and the social relations of everyday life (Oliver 1996, Shakespeare 2006, Gilroy et al. 2013).

Finally, market-based biomedicine plays a negligible role in contributing to the advancement of health equity. As we have seen most starkly in relation to the United States, biomedicine is one of the key social processes involved in the making of health inequity. Health care costs can actually create poverty and contribute to social division and marginalisation, particularly when health care is chronically under resourced (Marmot et al. 2012). Despite the size of government contributions to health care expenditure in some high-income countries, many people continue to face ruinous or catastrophic out-of-pocket healthcare expenses that result in the financial collapse of families (Clarke et al. 2011, Ehrle and Cleveland 2010, Yoon et al. 2011). Upwards of 100 million people are pushed into poverty yearly through the catastrophic household health costs that result from payments for access to services (Xu et al. 2007). The provision of subsidised health service arrangements delivered through formal employment or through tax deductions or tax incentives, while ensuring middle-class access to health care, has little or no effect on access to health care by the poor. These include people without paid employment or who have levels of income below the taxation threshold and people in informal employment or without citizenship, including refugees, guest workers and migrant workers. These are population groups at greatest risk of morbidity at the bottom of the social gradient, whose marginality may even extend to exclusion from official health statistics (Gideon 2013, Vearey 2013). Yet, the international evidence is unequivocal: public health-care spending has a greater positive effect on mortality among poor people than their more affluent counterparts (Bidani and Ravaillon 1997, Gupta, Verhoven and Tiongson 2003, Wagstaff and van Doorslaer 2003).

Certainly outside the United States, many global metropolitan states and their affiliates have intervened to address some of the barriers that market-based biomedicine poses for health equity. Pre-payment methods of financing through general taxation and/or mandatory universal health insurance provide more equitable health care and health (Gilson et al. 2007). Wealthy OECD countries in which governments have made these kinds of policy and funding interventions into market provision of health care clearly demonstrate such an effect. Nevertheless, as the WHO's Commission on the Social Determinants of Health (2008: 94) has pointed out, 'the inverse care law (Tudor-Hart 1971), in which the poor consistently gain less from health services than the better off, is visible in every country across the globe.'

Health care in the Global South: Financial impoverishment and biomedical markets

The inverse care law, however, does not operate simply according to dynamics of social inequality within countries. The inverse care law has gone global and operates as an integral feature of the dynamics of global division. As we have seen, health care accounts for one-tenth of the world's GDP, the lion's share of which goes to less than one-tenth of the world's population – namely those in the global metropole and their affiliates in the Global South. Yet, as the evidence presented throughout this book has disclosed, the 'burden' of illness, disability and mortality weighs far more heavily on the global periphery, especially in sub-Saharan Africa and South Asia.

The WHO's *Closing the Gap* report comments that 'people who are poor in low- and middle-income countries may have little or no access to health care' and 'over half a million women giving birth die each year with little or no access to maternity care' (CSDH 2008: 94). These comments apply most directly to sub-Saharan Africa and South Asia. The profile of health care organisation across these regions, however, is highly variable, especially between sub-Saharan Africa and India. In the former, state health expenditure is more prevalent and generally 'redistributive', meaning that most of it does reach those in the lowest-income categories (Chu, Davoodi and Gupta 2004, Kida and Mackintosh 2005). Uganda, for example, abolished user fees at public sector health facilities in March 2001, with the exception of private wards. Utilisation of health services increased immediately and dramatically. The poor particularly benefited from the removal of fees, with health services utilisation increasing from 58 to 70 per cent in the case of the poorest quintile and from 80 to 85 per cent for those in the richest quintile (Balabanova 2007, O'Donnell et al. 2007 cited in Gilson et al. 2007: 105–6). However,

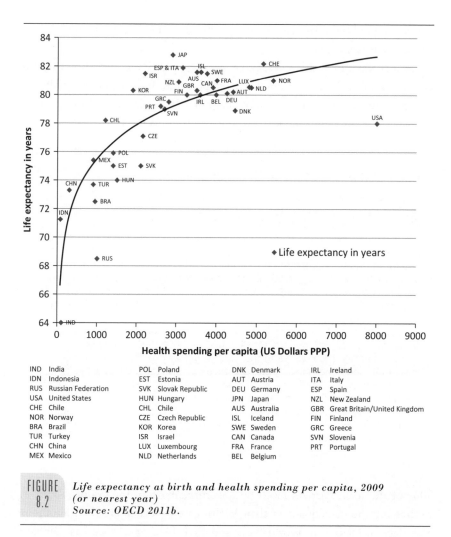

IND	India	POL	Poland	DNK	Denmark	IRL	Ireland
IDN	Indonesia	EST	Estonia	AUT	Austria	ITA	Italy
RUS	Russian Federation	SVK	Slovak Republic	DEU	Germany	ESP	Spain
USA	United States	HUN	Hungary	JPN	Japan	NZL	New Zealand
CHE	Chile	CHL	Chile	AUS	Australia	GBR	Great Britain/United Kingdom
NOR	Norway	CZE	Czech Republic	ISL	Iceland	FIN	Finland
BRA	Brazil	KOR	Korea	SWE	Sweden	GRC	Greece
TUR	Turkey	ISR	Israel	CAN	Canada	SVN	Slovenia
CHN	China	LUX	Luxembourg	FRA	France	PRT	Portugal
MEX	Mexico	NLD	Netherlands	BEL	Belgium		

FIGURE 8.2 *Life expectancy at birth and health spending per capita, 2009 (or nearest year)*
Source: OECD 2011b.

throughout sub-Saharan Africa there is certainly no primary health care and universal health coverage of the kind that prevails in Costa Rica and Cuba.

The situation is rather different in South Asia's most populous country, India. There is extremely limited public expenditure on health care. In fact, its 2012 rate of 4 per cent of GDP was on average less than half the rate of its African state counterparts, and among the lowest in the world. This was despite the fact that India's economy was ranked 10th-largest in the world by GDP in the same year (World Bank 2014f). Figure 8.2, charting overall health spending per capita (and life expectancy) among a number of countries in 2009, shows India's as the very lowest.

At the same time, however, India supports a thriving diversity of health care markets, including corporatised biomedicine. Its clientele not only includes members of the Indian upper class but increasingly wealthy 'medical tourists' from both high and low-income countries (Whittaker 2008).

Medical tourism 21st-century, Indian style

'Mediescapes India', according to its own website description, is a 'medical tourism services operator'. It provides the prospective client with a range of hospitals, procedures and medical conditions from which to choose. Mediescapes India puts the client in touch with the preferred hospitals and provides an 'international patient' assistant – or minder – to accompany the patient to medical appointments, and to arrange transfers to the hotel or resort of choice for recuperation. Most websites advertise the money to be saved in using their services. 'One site ... states, "Medical treatment in USA equals to [sic] a tour in India [plus] medical treatment in India [plus] savings"' (Whittaker 2008: 80).

Apollo Hospital Enterprises is the largest corporation offering hospital treatment for foreign tourists, totalling 60 000 in 2001–04. Owning 13 hospitals and managing a further 20, as well as 10 clinics, with more than 4000 beds, the Apollo group exemplifies corporatised global health care. It operates out of Sri Lanka, Muscat, Dubai, India, Nepal, Tanzania and Bangladesh, advertising its 'expertise in "super-specialties" of cardiology and neurosurgery, as well as transplants, orthopaedics, cancer treatment, and ... a range of other services, including IVF clinics, preventive health checks, and medical imaging' (Whittaker 2008: 280).

One of the main barriers faced by governments from the Global South in addressing the inadequacy of their health care provision are the limitations they face in relation to World Bank and IMF funding. As we have already seen, such global metropolitan financial institutions impose severe strictures on the internal economic governance of countries to whom they lend money for 'development'. This has been especially pronounced in sub-Saharan Africa since the 1960s and 1970s (Havnevik 1987) Many states in this region have been pressured to adopt neo-liberal approaches to health care and welfare provision, restricting their development of primary health care and universal health coverage – what some describe as 'enhanced scarcity' of health care (Streefland 2005).

Finally, and possibly the most pressing barrier that health care systems in the global periphery face, is access to skilled health providers. According to the

WHO's landmark report on the global health workforce, *Working Together for Health*: 'at the heart of each and every health system, the workforce is central to advancing health' (2006: xv). Yet, 57 countries throughout the world have so few 'human resources for health' that they have been identified by the WHO as being in 'crisis'. Not surprisingly, the region most harshly affected is sub-Saharan Africa. 'With only 3 percent of the world's health workers but 24 percent of the world's burden of disease, the more than 50 countries that comprise the region are expected to suffer a catastrophic decline in the survival rates of women in childbirth and children in early infancy ... OECD countries, by contrast, are not facing critical shortages' (Schofield 2012b: 57). The WHO (2006) estimates that a further 4.5 million health workers are needed to redress and prevent the crisis.

One of the single biggest drivers of this crisis is what some have called the 'brain drain' in health care from the global periphery (Iredale 2012: 19). Doctors, nurses, midwives and other skilled health workers, trained mainly at public expense, have been leaving their low and middle-income countries of origin in droves. They search for better lives with higher pay and better working conditions, and are usually successful in their quest. The reason they do so is because many high-income states have health workforce shortages as a result of severe problems in staff retention (Iredale 2012, Schofield 2012b). Such problems indicate serious deficiencies in health system organisation and management (Schofield 2009, Kuhlmann and Annandale 2012). Yet, instead of addressing the sources of the problems, high-income countries have been actively recruiting overseas health workers from precisely the countries facing potentially catastrophic shortages. Some have described this approach by global metropolitan states and their affiliates as 'health workforce poaching', with many raising concerns about the ethics and 'sustainability' of such an approach (Ransome and Sampford 2012). Despite these concerns, the health workforce policies and practices of the privileged world show no sign of retreat from global poaching.

Conclusions

There are few other social institutions that attract such universal approval and support as health care. In contemporary times, doctors, nurses and others involved in its provision command widespread social recognition. And often for good reason. Health care can mean the difference between life and death, and relief from pain and suffering, both physical and mental. Yet, as this chapter has explained, some kinds of health care are far more effective in promoting health and reducing health inequalities than others. It all depends on how health care is socially organised and how it works as a social process. Basically, a global division structures the organisation and provision of health care throughout the world. The global metropole and its affiliates spend the lion's share of the world's health expenditure. They deliver health services and medical goods mainly through markets dominated by global corporations and professionally controlled, high-tech biomedicine that focuses on individual organic dysfunction and cure. State processes work hand-in-hand with health care markets, offering large subsidies – in differing amounts, according to national health policy – to support market distribution. Access to health care consequently varies among the rich countries of the OECD depending on the extent to which governments fund their citizens' health coverage. Health results vary concomitantly, with disparities greatest in the United States even though it spends the highest proportion of GDP of all OECD countries on health.

The Global South discloses a more varied pattern of health care organisation, funding and outcomes than its wealthy counterparts. Sub-Saharan Africa confronts a 'crisis' in health care with limited state resource allocation available to meet even the most basic provision and the relentless exodus of its health workforce to the Global North. Meanwhile, Indian public investment in health care is among the lowest in the world despite the size of its economy, with much of its highly skilled health workforce engaged in high-tech medical provision to paying customers, both national and international. Health outcomes in sub-Saharan Africa and South Asia (including India), as documented in previous chapters, reflect two main features related to state approaches to health care: financial impoverishment and relinquishment to the market of service distribution. Yet, others in the Global South – notably Costa Rica and Cuba – have achieved health outcomes comparable to those of the Global North. At the heart of their success has been a number of factors, but resistance to the dictates of international financial institutions to curb public health care and universal health coverage has been central. So, too, has been the institution of a primary health care system integrated with rural and urban community development. Medicine has played a key role also, but not on a fee-for-service basis or as central decision makers in determining the organisation and delivery of health care.

It is evident, then, that health care has become increasingly commodified or dominated by markets in terms of its organisation and distribution and, with this, a growing emphasis on high-tech biomedicine at the expense of primary health care. As such, health care can be understood as an industry. Various stakeholders have been involved in driving this development, creating a major disparity in access to health care between the world's rich minority and its marginalised majority. The most notable among these include international financial institutions, medical or health care corporations, pharmaceutical and other manufacturers of health care and medical products, health insurance companies, and medical professional associations (Bond and Dor 2003, Homedes and Ugalde 2005, Lister 2007).

From a sociological perspective, health care operates like many other global corporate industries, subject to the major dynamics of social division and its inequitable health outcomes, both within and between countries. Because there are a number of complex *concepts* critical to understanding these dynamics, we summarise them in this concluding paragraph. First is *global division*, as discussed in previous chapters. The social dynamics associated with it exert enormous influence in shaping the *social relations of health care* that prevail within and between countries; that is, solidaristic or *cooperative* versus market-based or *commodified*, or sometimes on a continuum between the two. Based in the Global North, the internationally dominant pattern is market-based and driven by *biomedical discourse and practice*. These dynamics are integrally related to those associated with the *division of labour* in health care, primarily *professionalisation* and *medical dominance*. Here, *class* and *gender* are critical. As a key player in the process, the *state* participates in a number of ways. One is as *regulator* of the kind of social relations of health care that prevail, and the *legitimation* of those who can provide and manage it. The state also participates through its *re-distributive* actions associated with health insurance and health system funding policies. Among the wealthy OECD countries, those with more re-distributive health policies achieve greater health equity in terms of health outcomes. In some parts of the Global South, such as Costa Rica and Cuba, the state has challenged the globally dominant pattern of health care, provoking vigorous opposition from powerful international financial institutions that support individualised, corporatised and marketised public governance and that promotes commodified health care arrangements.

Questions for discussion

1 What do you understand by the 'social relations of health care'?
2 What is primary health care and how can it be described in terms of the social relations of health care?
3 How does primary health care improve health outcomes and advance health equity?

4   What is market-based health care and how is its pervasiveness linked to global division and corporate growth?

5   What is biomedicine and how does it differ from primary health care?

6   What role does the state play in relation to commodified health care and biomedicine in the Global North and its affiliates?

7   What is medical dominance?

8   How is the professionalisation of medicine related to the social dynamics of class, gender and the state in the Global North and its affiliates?

9   Why does market-based health care in some wealthy OECD countries produce more equitable health outcomes than others?

10   What are some of the main adverse health effects of the dominance of market-based biomedicine in wealthy OECD countries?

11   How does the dominance of market-based biomedicine adversely affect health care and health in the Global South?

12   To what extent is economic growth in the Global South imperative for the development of better health care and improved health outcomes?

Epilogue

A common response to sociology is: 'What do I do with this?' (Russell and Schofield 1986: 203). Physical scientists' research can often be taken up for 'practical' purposes, such as providing cures and treatments for disease and injury. A sociological approach offers no comparable technical solution – no 'magic bullet'. Not that sociology has a singular mission. In its comparatively short history, it has had many purposes. In this book, its 'project' has been inspired and shaped by international policy and research development in health: the social determinants of health. As Chapter 1 explained, the 'social determinants of health' has become a globally influential approach to understanding and responding to social inequalities and health disparities, both within countries and globally. Pioneered by the WHO, it has entered the lexicon of health policy makers, health practitioners, researchers and social movements. It has generated a seismic shift in global awareness of the inter-connectedness of the differentiated health fates of the planet's peoples, and of the injustices that accompany them. Its central 'take-home' message is that health disparities are of our making and, therefore, can be un-made. What's more, the problem does not lie with insufficient global resources. Rather, the problem and its solution are located squarely within the realm of human society; in particular, 'social factors' associated with how we live, work and grow.

However, as this book has proposed throughout, identifying solutions to problems from a scientific perspective requires knowledge and understanding based on systematic and rigorous analysis of how things work, not simply on the cataloguing and measurement of the recurrent patterns involved. Within social science, the latter prevails very widely, often drawing on large databases and statistical analyses of them. This is a critically important task, especially in relation to global health. Yet, 'un-making' human social problems demands knowledge and understanding of the barriers and opportunities for the kinds of human action required. Enter sociology.

In sociology, as in all the social sciences, there is no global consensus on 'the social' and how to study and understand it. Animating and informing the approach developed in this book is a tradition that views the social as an accomplishment of human *practice,* and one subject to complex dynamics that vary historically and in different places throughout the world. In addressing the un-making of social inequality and health disparity, such an approach has compelling relevance, highlighted by its distinction from other influential 'sociologies'. At the heart of the sociology advanced in this book is the idea that the social is dynamic rather than static. Static approaches, by contrast, often seek to capture and understand the social by mapping social space in terms of categories that are like slots into which groups of people are located. The study of class, for example, has been very much influenced by such an approach. Class 'systems' are represented as an hierarchy of steps or levels across which people are distributed according to characteristics they possess, such as income level, educational qualifications, occupational rank, recreational activities, residential location, car ownership and so on. How the various levels came to exist in the first place, and how and why they continue to do so, remain outside the frame of knowledge and understanding. Since such approaches exclude from investigation and analysis how the hierarchy itself is generated – or how it works – the possibility for examining how it might be undone or dismantled is precluded. Given the nature of the problem of social inequality and global health disparity, a dynamic and critical sociology is imperative.

The making and unmaking of health inequity as a dynamic social – and political – process

In adopting a dynamic lens, then, the central proposition of this book is that health inequity itself is a social process – something people do and that is done to them through social practice and the relationships through which it is enacted. This process operates on both a national and global basis – in local settings, within and between institutions, at national levels, among countries and between them. Yet, no matter where or when, social practice is patterned or structured, so there are parameters or boundaries we encounter in participating in the process. The social is complex but it does not endlessly repeat the same patterns. Those that are enduring, pervasive and influential, both within and beyond national borders, are dominant structures of practice – such as class, gender, ethnicity, indigeneity and the state. They do not all *necessarily* generate social inequality. In fact, it is only class, in partnership with global division, that is intrinsically divisive. Gender, ethnicity, indigeneity and the state can work as sources of social difference and diversity. However, their present-day combination makes access to health unevenly distributed because it renders access to the social resources needed for health unequal. These resources are material, symbolic and agentic. As we have seen from the evidence, they enable people individually and collectively to participate with others in making lives for themselves over which they can exercise direction and influence, and from which they can derive material security and social recognition – as valued members of the communities in which they live and work, and through respect for their rights as individuals. Social relations and practices that distribute social resources along these lines produce more equitable health outcomes. It hardly looks like the stuff of which utopias are made. Yet, the large-scale inequality in social resource distribution, together with the relentlessness with which social dynamics generate it, make the conditions for health equity *appear* utopian.

The normalisation of social inequality and the exercise of power through which it has been achieved have been insidiously successful, as this book has demonstrated. One of the most powerful mechanisms involved in the process has been the sheer volubility and repetition of discourses, such as those associated with the propagation of neo-liberalism, suggesting that the interests of the vast majority are those of a very small minority. Such a proposition – arguably one of the most enduring of ideologies – has attracted collective opposition and organised resistance over a very long time and in many diverse locations, as we have seen throughout this book. Progress towards greater social equality and health equity has only advanced on the back of critique and political contestation of dominant minority interests whose benefits are gained at the expense of the majority.

This resistance continues into the 21st century. The 'communications revolution', for instance, has opened up innovative electronic possibilities for developing regional and global solidarities and interventions into the routine enactment of social inequality and its health effects. Such an approach can be understood as a *tactics* of contestation that consistently challenges and resists prevailing ways of thinking and doing things that perpetuate inequality and injustice. Its most visible effect has been to demonstrate that the dominant representational or discursive universe does not 'have it all its own way' – so much so that in some instances those engaged in such contestation have been denounced as threats to 'national security' by various powers of the Global North. The 'new communications' and its subversive practitioners undoubtedly operate as a source of 'counter hegemony', albeit in anarchic and disorganised ways.

Any attempt to mount effective international opposition to the powerhouse of global division and its inequitable effects on health, however, demands more than disorganised resistance. A *strategic* approach characterised by coordinated regional and international engagement is critical. Yet, the chances of such an engagement in successfully challenging the enormous disparities in resource distribution and control require participation by national states and major global institutions. Clearly, they are presently a major part of 'the problem', as this book has explained. But because of the critical role they play in rule and governance, especially in relation to control of resources and their distribution, they are absolutely foundational to any strategic intervention to advance social and health equity. Central to the success of such an intervention, of course, is *majority* popular support and participation – or 'buy in'. After all, it is the overwhelming majority of the world's peoples who stand to benefit most by such an intervention, and unless they are actively a part of it, they can be too readily mobilised by forces of reaction against it, as the past 100 years have so amply demonstrated. Here, states are also crucial because of their control over much of the machinery for popular participation.

As previously mentioned in this book, such machinery includes political parties and state-based political processes offering opportunities for participation that can contribute to the advancement of social equity. This machinery encompasses *employment* in state and other state-funded organisations (such as the large sector of non-government, not-for-profit agencies that depends heavily on state funding in Australia) engaged in policy making, and the development, delivery and management of programs and services to reduce social inequalities and to promote health equity. There are, however, numerous other avenues for such participation in 'civil society'. Many of these interact with and shape the state's operations. Membership of social movements, for instance, provides opportunities for organised participation in campaigns and activities designed to challenge and change the processes responsible for the systematic production and reproduction of social and health inequity. Though they focus on distinctive social 'constituencies' with specific interests, social movements such as the trade union movement, the women's movement, the Indigenous rights movement, the environment movement, the disability movement and the gay rights movement, all offer opportunities to participate in action to redress social and health inequity. The number of organisations they incorporate is very large, and criteria for membership are designed to maximise inclusion rather than exclusivity.

Though now a well-worn cliché emanating from the environmental movement, the mantra to 'think globally, act locally' remains a useful slogan in building popular support and framing action for change. As the analysis developed in this book suggests, the politics of the social dynamics involved in the creation of social inequality and health disparity operate at multiple levels of social organisation and practice. There are thus many points for organised and legitimate 'local' intervention. All such action, however, usually demands *collective participation* and cooperative engagement with others. Just as significant are knowledge and understanding of the social dynamics involved in producing and reproducing 'the problem'. As this book has explained in relation to health inequity and its social determinants, knowledge and understanding of 'the social' that is informed by static categories such as 'social factors' cannot illuminate how the social actually works. As we have learnt, it operates in specific and complex ways in determining health inequity. Such knowledge and understanding serve a central practical purpose in relation to 'the problem' of health inequity. They are fundamental for formulating strategies and actions to address and redress it. Failure to develop and operationalise such knowledge and understanding poses formidable threats to the survival of large swathes of the world's peoples. The spread of HIV/AIDS in sub-Saharan Africa, for example, has been attributable to several dynamics, but one of the most damaging has been the reluctance of policy makers, especially at an international level, to invest in a systematic investigation of the complex social processes operating in the spread of HIV/AIDS, and identification of the barriers and opportunities for effective social interventions. A similar situation has been developing in relation to the spread of the Ebola virus that has already been responsible for the death of thousands people in West Africa and is predicted to kill many more. European disease modelling suggests that its international spread is inevitable, with some European countries, including the United Kingdom, at highest risk.

While the Global South has shouldered most of the health burden associated with HIV/AIDS, the wealthy populations of the Global North have not been immune. HIV/AIDS, for instance, has exacted a significant death toll in all the major high-income countries. A similar scenario may prevail in relation to Ebola. Yet, a further and arguably more formidable health threat emanating in the Global South, but likely to have a significant effect on a number of wealthy countries, especially Australia, Japan, New Zealand and the United States, is that predicted to result from the social and health effects of catastrophic weather events associated with climate change, as previously discussed. Such effects will include very high rates of mortality, infectious disease and injury, and the mass destruction of habitat and social infrastructure that will generate mass starvation and huge numbers of displaced people and refugees, mainly from South Asia, South-east Asia and the Pacific Islands. The capacity of the Global North to withstand such threats will depend on a range of public responses, undoubtedly including 'border protection' and military action, if the prevailing Australian response is any indication of possible reactions among wealthy nation states. But if the wealthy nations of the Global North want to protect and secure the health of their citizens on a sustainable and durable basis, effective intervention will require a far-sighted approach, focused on *preventive* action. As this book has argued, no such action is possible without recognising and understanding the social dynamics that determine social and health inequity – both locally and globally. Against such a backdrop, knowledge of the social and how to deal with the threats it creates for our shared survival is certainly power. But only if that knowledge is further developed and disseminated, and widely mobilised across both the Global North and Global South as a basis for action. Clearly, this is a political process – knowledge and understanding of which are also critical, but that is another complex story.

References

Abdool, S.N., Garcia-Moreno, C. and Amin, A. (2012) 'Gender equality and international health policy', In E. Kuhlmann and E. Annandale (eds) *The Palgrave Handbook of Gender and Healthcare*, 2nd edn, pp. 36–55, Houndmills, Basingstoke: Palgrave Macmillan.

Aboriginal Healing Foundation (2003) *Fetal Alcohol Syndrome Among Aboriginal People in Canada: Review and Analysis of the Intergenerational Links to Residential Schools*, Ottawa: Aboriginal Healing Foundation.

Acevedo-Garcia, D., Osypuk, T.L., McArdle, N. and Williams, D.R. (2008) 'Toward a policy-relevant analysis of geographic and racial/ethnic disparities in child health', *Health Affairs*, 27(2): 321–33.

Achebe, C. (1985) 'Civil peace', In C. Achebe and C.L. Innes (eds) *African Short Stories*, pp. 29–34, London, Ibadan and Nairobi: Heinemann.

Adi, H. (2012) *Africa and the Transatlantic Slave Trade*. Accessed at: www.bbc.co.uk/history/british/abolition/africa_article_01.shtml, 12 April 2013.

Adiga, A. (2008) *The White Tiger*, London: Atlantic Books.

Adriaanse, J. and Schofield, T. (2013) 'Analysing gender dynamics in sport governance: A new regimes-based approach', *Sport Management Review*, 16(4): 498–513.

Agency for Health Care Research and Quality (2012) *2011 National Healthcare Disparities Report*, Rockville, MD. Accessed at: www.ahrq.gov/research/findings/nhqrdr/nhdr11/index.html, 15 January 2014.

Agudelo-Suárez, A.A., Ronda-Pérez, E., and Benavides, F.G. (2011) 'Occupational health', In B. Rechel, P. Mladovsky, W. Devillé, B. Rijks, R. Petrova-Benedict and M. McKee (eds) *Migration and Health in the European Union*, pp. 155–68, Maidenhead: Open University Press and McGraw-Hill.

Alcorso, C. and Schofield, T. (1991) *The National Non-English Speaking Background Women's Health Strategy*, Canberra: AGPS.

Alderete, E., Erickson, P., Kaplan, C. and Perez-Stable, E. (2010) 'Ceremonial tobacco use in the Andes: Implications for smoking prevention among Indigenous youth', *Anthropological Medicine*, 17(1): 27–39.

Alderete, E., Haswell, M., Ring, I., Waldon, J., Clark, W., Whetung, V., Kinnon, D., Graham, C., Chino, M., La Valley and Sadana, R. (1999) *The Health of Indigenous Peoples*, Geneva: World Health Organization. Accessed at: http://apps.who.int/iris/handle/10665/65609, 5 September 2014.

Allsop, J. (2006) 'Medical dominance in a changing world: The UK case', *Health Sociology Review*, 15: 444–57.

Altman, J. (2001) ' "Mutual obligation", the CDEP scheme, and development: Prospects in remote Australia', In F. Morphy and W. Sanders (eds) *The Indigenous Welfare Economy and the CDEP Scheme*, Research Monograph No. 20, pp. 125–34, Canberra: Centre for Aboriginal Economic Policy Research, Australian National University.

Annandale, E. (2003) 'Gender and health status: Does biology matter?', In S. Williams, L. Birke and G. Bendelow (eds) *Debating Biology: Social Reflections on Health*, pp. 84–95, London: Routledge.

Anthony, T. (2004) *The Ghost of Feudalism: Aboriginal Land and Labour Dependencies in the Northern Australian Cattle Industry*, Sydney: University of Sydney Press.

Anthony, T. and Cuneen, C. (eds) *The Critical Criminology Companion*, pp. 30–42, Leichhardt, NSW: Hawkins Press.

Anttonen, A. and Meagher, G. (2013) 'Mapping marketisation: Concepts and goals', In G. Meagher and M. Szebehely (eds) *Marketisation in Nordic Eldercare: A Research Report on Legislation, Oversight, Extent and Consequences*, Stockholm Studies in Social Work 30, pp. 13–22, Stockholm: Department of Social Work, Stockholm University.

Archer, J. and Lloyd. B. (1982) *Sex and Gender*, Ringwood, Vic.: Penguin.

Arneil, B. (1994) 'Trade, plantations and property: John Locke and the economic defence of colonialism', *Journal of the History of Ideas*, 55(4): 591–609.

Arnold, J.M., Brys, B., Heady, C., Johansson, A., Schwellnus, C. and Vartia, L. (2011) 'Tax policy for economic recovery and growth', *The Economic Journal*,121(550): F59–80.

Aron, R. (1965) *Main Currents in Sociological Thought*, Ringwood, Vic.: Penguin.

Astley, T. (1987) *It's Raining in Mango: Pictures from a Family Album*, Ringwood, Vic.: Penguin.

Atwall, A. and Caldwell, K. (2005) 'Do all health and social care professionals interact equally?: A study of interactions in multidisciplinary teams in the United Kingdom, *Scandinavian Journal of Caring Sciences*, 19(3): 268–73.

Austin-Broos, D. (2011) *A Different Inequality: The Politics of Debate About Remote Aboriginal Australia*, Sydney: Allen & Unwin.

Australian Bureau of Statistics (ABS) (2014) *Population Clock*. Accessed at: http://abs.gov.au/AUSSTATS/abs@.nsf/Web+Pages/Population+Clock?opendocument, 5 September 2014.

ABS (2013a) *Schools Australia*, Catalogue No. 4221.0. Accessed at: www.abs.gov.au, 6 May 2014.

ABS (2013b) *Prisoners in Australia: 2013*, Catalogue No. 4517.0. Accessed at: www.abs.gov.au, 6 May 2014.

ABS (2012a) *Employee Earnings and Hours Australia*, Catalogue No. 6306.0. Accessed at: http://www.abs.gov.au/ausstats/abs@.nsf/mf/6306.0/, 26 February 2014.

ABS (2012b) *Evolution of Australian Industry Year Book Australia*, Catalogue No. 1301.0. Accessed at: http://www.abs.gov.au/ausstats/abs@.nsf/mf/1301.0, 3 March 2014.

ABS (2011) Greater Darwin: People, *Census of Population and Housing 2011*. Accessed at: www.censusdata.abs.gov.au/census_services/getproduct/census/2011/quickstat/7GDAR?opendocument&navpos=220, 16 June 2014.

ABS (2010) *The Health and Welfare of Australia's Aboriginal and Torres Strait Islander Peoples*, Catalogue No. 4704.0. Accessed at: www.abs.gov.au, 6 May 2014.

ABS (2006) *Population Distribution, Aboriginal and Torres Strait Islander Australians*, Catalogue No. 4705.0. Accessed at: www.abs.gov.au./ausstats/abs@nsf, 6 March 2013.

Australian Human Rights and Equal Opportunity Commission (HREOC) (1997) *Bringing Them Home: The Stolen Children Report*, Canberra: HREOC.

Australian Human Rights Commission (2012) Independent Interim Report on CEDAW: Australian Human Rights Commission Report to the Committee on the Elimination of All Forms of Discrimination Against Women, Sydney. Accessed at: www.humanrights.gov.au/independent-interim-report-cedaw, 4 September 2014.

Australian Institute of Health and Welfare (AIHW) (2014) *Australia's Health 2014*, Canberra: AIHW. Accessed at: www.aihw.gov.au/publication-detail/?id=60129547205, 4 September 2014.

AIHW (2013a) 'Australian hospital statistics 2011–12', *Health Services*, Series 50. Catalogue No. HSE 134, Canberra: AIHW. Accessed at: www.aihw.gov.au/hospitals/#ahs, 26 June 2014.

AIHW (2013b) *Cancer in Aboriginal and Torres Strait Islander Peoples of Australia: An Overview*, Catalogue No. CAN 75, Canberra: AIHW.

AIHW (2013c) *Indigenous Health*, Canberra: AIHW. Accessed at: www.aihw.gov.au/indigenous-health, 6 March 2013.

AIHW (2012) *Older Australians at a Glance*, 4th edn, Canberra: AIHW. Accessed at www.aihw.gov.au/publication-detail/?id=6442468045&libID=6442468043, 27 June 2014.

AIHW (2011a) *The Health and Welfare of Australia's Aboriginal and Torres Strait Islander People: An Overview*, Catalogue No. IHW 42, Canberra: AIHW.

AIHW (2011b) *2010 National Drug Strategy Household Survey Report*, Catalogue No. PHE 145, Canberra: AIHW.

AIHW (2010) *Australia's Health 2010*. Canberra: AIHW. Accessed at: www.aihw.gov.au/ WorkArea/DownloadAsset.aspx?id=6442452955#Page=44, 9 February 2014.

AIHW (2008a) *The Health and Welfare of Australia's Aboriginal and Torres Strait Islander Peoples*, Catalogue No. IHW 21, Canberra: AIHW.

AIHW (2008b) *Cardiovascular Disease and its Associated Risk Factors in Aboriginal and Torres Strait Islander Peoples 2004–2005*, Catalogue No. CVD 41, Canberra: AIHW.

Balabanova, D. (2007) 'Health sector reform and equity in transition', Paper prepared for the Health Systems Knowledge Network of the World Health Organization's Commission on Social Determinants of Health'. Cited in L. Gilson, J. Doherty, R. Lowenson and V. Francis, *Final Report of World Health Organization Knowledge Network on Health Systems of the World Health Organization Commission on the Social Determinants of Health*, London: Centre for Health Policy at the University of the Witwatersrand, South Africa, EQUINET and the Health Policy Unit of the London School of Hygiene and Tropical Medicine.

Bales, K. (2012) *Disposable People: New Slavery in the Global Economy* (3rd edn), Berkeley: University of California Press.

Barrett, M. and McIntosh, M. (1982) 'The "family wage"', In E. Whitelegg, M. Arnot, E. Bartels, V. Beechey, L. Birke, S. Himmelweit and D. Leonard (eds) *The Changing Experience of Women*, Oxford: Martin Robertson.

Barrett-Connor, E. (2013) 'Gender difference and disparities in all-case and coronary heart disease mortality: Epidemiological aspects', *Best Practice and Research: Clinical Endocrinology and Metabolism*, 27(4): 481–500.

Bartrip, P.W.J. and Burman, S.B. (1983) *The Wounded Soldiers of Industry: Industrial Compensation Policy 1833–1897*, Oxford: Clarendon Press.

Baum, F. (2008) *The New Public Health* (3rd edn), Melbourne: Oxford University Press.

Beaglehole, R., Epping-Jordan, J., Patel, V., Chopra, M., Ebrahim, D.M., Kidd, M. and Haines, A. (2008) 'Improving the prevention and management of chronic disease in low-income and middle-income countries: A priority for primary health care', *The Lancet*, 372(9642): 940–49.

Beck, U. (1992) *Risk Society: Towards a New Modernity*, Newbury Park: Sage.

Beck, U. and Beck-Gernsheim, E. (2002) *Individualization: Institutionalized Individualism and its Social and Political Consequences*, London: Sage.

Beilharz, P. (1991) 'Max Weber', In P. Beilharz (ed.) *Social Theory: A Guide to Central Thinkers*, pp. 224–30, North Sydney: Allen & Unwin.

Berman, M. (1988) *All That is Solid Melts into Air: The Experience of Modernity*, New York: Viking Penguin.

Bhopal, R.S. (2007) *Ethnicity, Race, and Health in Multicultural Societies: Foundations for Better Epidemiology, Public Health and Health Care*, Oxford: Oxford University Press.

Bhutta, Z., Ali, S., Cousens, S., Ali, M., Haider, B., Rizvi, A., Okong, P., Bhutta, S. and Black, R.E (2008) 'Interventions to address maternal, newborn, and child survival: what difference can integrated primary health care strategies make?' *The Lancet*, 372: 972–89.

Bidani, B. and Ravaillon, M. (1997) 'Decomposing social indicators using distributional data', *Journal of Econometrics*, 77(1): 125–39.

Bird, C.E., Lang, M.E. and Rieker, P.P. (2012) 'Changing gendered patterns of morbidity and mortality', In E. Kuhlmann and E. Annandale (eds) *The Palgrave Handbook of Gender and Healthcare*, 2nd edn, pp. 145–61, Houndmills, Basingstoke, Hampshire: Palgrave Macmillan.

Birrell, B. and Healy, E. (2013) *The Impact of Recent Immigration on the Australian Workforce*, Centre for Population and Urban Research, Monash University. Accessed at: http://artsonline. monash.edu.au/cpur/files/2013/02/Immigration_review__Feb-2013.pdf, 4 September 2014.

Blackburn, E. and Epel, E.S. (2012) 'Telomeres and adversity: Too toxic to ignore', *Nature*, 490(7419): 169–71, 10 October.

Blackburn, R. (2012) 'Slavery, emancipation and human rights', In K.E. Tunstall (ed.) *Self-Evident Truths?: Human Rights and the Enlightenment*, pp. 137–56, New York and London: Bloomsbury.

Blakey, M.L. (1999) 'Scientific racism and the biological concept of race', *Literature and Psychology*, 45(1/2): 29–43.

Blane, D. (2006) 'The life course, the social gradient, and health', In M. Marmot and R. Wilkinson (eds) *Social Determinants of Health*, 2nd edn, Oxford: Oxford University Press.

Bloom, M. (1995) *Understanding Sickle Cell Disease*, Jackson: University Press of Mississippi.

Boas, F. (1912) 'Changes in the bodily form of descendants of immigrants', *American Anthropologist*, 14(3): 530–62.

Bond, P. and Dor, G. (2003) 'Uneven health outcomes and political resistance under residual neoliberalism in Africa', *International Journal of Health Services*, 33(3): 607–30.

Booth, A.L., Leigh, A. and Varganova, E. (2012) 'Does ethnic discrimination vary across minority groups? Evidence from a field experiment', *Oxford Bulletin of Economics and Statistics*, 74(4): 547–73.

Borchorst, A. and Siim, B. (2008) 'Woman-friendly policies and state feminism: Theorizing Scandinavian gender equality', *Feminist Theory*, 9(2): 207–24.

Bourdieu, P. and Wacquant, L. (1992) *An Invitation to Reflexive Sociology*, Cambridge: Polity Press.

Boysen, N., Fliedner, M. and Scholl, A. (2007) 'A classification of assembly line balancing problems', *European Journal of Operational Research*, 183(2): 674–93.

Bradfield, S. (2005) 'White picket fence or Trojan horse? The debate over communal land ownership of Indigenous land and individual land and individual wealth creation', *Land, Rights, Laws: Issues of Native Title*, 3(3): 1–11.

Branch, J.N. (2011) 'Mapping the sovereign state: Cartographic technology, political authority, and systemic change', University of California, Berkeley. Accessed at: http://gradworks.umi.com/34/69/3469226.html, 5 September 2014.

Brilmayer, L. and Klein, N. (2001) 'Land and sea: Two sovereignty regimes in search of a common denominator', *NYUJ of International Law and Politics*, 33: 703–6.

Brockerhoff, M., and Hewett, P. (2000) 'Inequality of child mortality among ethnic groups in Sub-Saharan Africa', *Bulletin of the World Health Organization*, 78(1): 30–41.

Broome, R. (2010) *Aboriginal Australians: A History Since 1788*, 4th edn, Sydney: Allen & Unwin.

Brown, T.M., Cueto, M. and Fee, E. (2006) 'The transition from "international" to "global" public health in the world', *Historia, Cience, Saude Manguinhos*, 13(3): 623–47 (article in Portuguese).

Brownlee, S. (2012) 'The scandal of "Pharmapayola"', *Time*, 30 January. Accessed at: http://ideas.time.com/2012/01/30/the-latest-big-pharma-scandal/?iid=op-article-latest, 14 January 2014.

Bryceson, D.F. (2010) 'Sub-Saharan Africa's vanishing peasantries and the spectre of a global food crisis', In F. Magdoff and B. Tokar (eds) *Agriculture and Food in Crisis: Crisis, Resistance and Renewal*, New York: Monthly Review Press, pp. 69–84.

Burawoy, M. (2000) 'Marxism after communism', *Theory and Society*, 29: 151–74.

Burgess, C.P., Johnston, F.H., Bowman, D.M.J.S. and Whitehead, P.J. (2005) 'Healthy country: healthy people? Exploring the health benefits of Indigenous natural resource management', *Australian and New Zealand Journal of Public Health*, 29(2): 117–22.

Busfield, J. (2012) 'Gender and mental health', In E. Kuhlmann and E. Annandale (eds) *The Palgrave Handbook of Gender and Healthcare*, 2nd edn, pp. 192–208, Houndmills, Basingstoke, Hampshire: Palgrave Macmillan.

Calladine, C.R., Drew, H.R., Luisi, B.F. and Travers, A. (2004) *Understanding DNA: The Molecule and How it Works*, 3rd edn, San Diego: Academic Press, Elsiever Science and Technology Books.

Campbell, E.G., Rao, S.R., DesRoches, C.M., Iezzoni, L.I., Vogeli, C., Bolcic-Jankovic D. and Miralles, P.D. (2010) 'Physician professionalism and changes in physician-industry relationships from 2004 to 2009', *Archives of Internal Medicine*, 170(20): 1820–6.

Canadian Partnership Against Cancer (2011) *First Nations, Inuit and Métis Action Plan on Cancer Control*. Accessed at: www.partnershipagainstcancer.ca/priorities/first-nations-inuit-metis-cancer-control/, 1 May 2014.

Carneiro, R.L. (1994) 'A theory of the origin of the state: Traditional theories of state origins are considered and rejected in favor of a new ecological hypothesis', In J.A. Hall (ed.) *The State: Critical Concepts*, pp. 1–43, London: Routledge.

Casper, M., Denny, C., Coolidge, J., Williams, G., Crowell, A., Galloway, J. and Cobb, N. (2005) *Atlas of Heart Disease and Stroke Among American Indians and Alaska Natives*, Atlanta: US Department of Health and Human Services, Centers for Disease Control and Prevention and Indian Health Service.

Centers for Disease Control and Prevention and The Merck Company Foundation (2007) *The State of Aging and Health in America*, Whitehouse Station, NJ: The Merck Company Foundation. Accessed at: www.cdc.gov/aging, 4 September 2014.

Chandra, A. (2009) 'Who you are and where you live: Race and the geography of healthcare', *Medical Care*, 47(2): 135–7.

Chang, J. (1991) *Wild Swans: Three Daughters of China*, London: Flamingo, HarperCollins.

Choo, H.Y. and Ferree, M.M. (2010) 'Practising intersectionality in sociological research: A critical analysis of inclusions, interactions, and institutions in the study of inequalities', *Sociological Theory*, 28(2): 129–49.

Chu, K.Y., Davoodi H. and Gupta S. (2004) 'Income distribution, tax and government spending policies in developing countries', In G.A. Cornia (ed.) *Inequality, Growth and Poverty in an Era of Liberalisation and Structural Adjustment*, Oxford University Press: Oxford. Cited in M. Mackintosh, K. Mensah, L. Henry and M. Rowson (2006) 'Aid, restitution and international fiscal redistribution in health care: Implications of health professionals' migration', *Journal of International Development*, 18: 757–70.

Claessen, H.J.M. and Skalnik, P. (1978) 'The early state: Theories and hypothesis', In H.J.M Claessen and P. Skalnik (eds) *The Early State*, The Hague: Mouton.

Clarke, A.E. and Shim, J. (2011). 'Medicalization and biomedicalization revisited: Technoscience and transformations of health, illness and American medicine', In B.A. Pescosolido, J.K. Martin, J.D. McLeod and A. Rogers (eds) *Handbook of the Sociology of Health, Illness: Blueprint for the 21st Century*, pp. 173–99, New York: Springer.

Clarke, C.R., Soukup, J., Govindarajulu, U., Rien, H.E., Tovar, D.A. and Johnson, P.A. (2011) 'Lack of access due to costs remains a problem for some in Massachusetts despite the State's health reforms', *Health Affairs*, 30(2): 247–55.

Claude, G., Margaret, M., Marie-France, G., Ravi, B., Loh, V. and Loh, S. (2005) *Projections of the Aboriginal Populations, Canada: Provinces and Territories*, Statistics Catalogue No. 91–547, Ottawa: Statistics Canada.

Clegg, S.R. (2006) 'Bureaucracy and public sector governmentality', In G. Ritzer (ed.) *The Blackwell Encyclopaedia of Sociology*, pp. 376–8, Malden, MA: Blackwell.

Coburn, D., Torrance, G.N. and Kaufert, J. (1983) 'Medical dominance in Canada in historical perspective: The rise and fall of medicine', *The International Journal of Health Services*, 13(3): 407–32.

Cockerham, W.C. (2005) 'Healthy lifestyle theory and the convergence of agency and structure', *Journal of Health and Social Behaviour*, 46(1): 51–67.

Cohen, A. (1999) *The Mental Health of Indigenous Peoples: An International Overview*, Geneva: Nations for Mental Health, Department of Mental Health, World Health Organization.

Collinson, D.L. and Hearn, J. (2009) 'Men, diversity at work, and diversity management', In M. Ozbilgin (ed.) *Equality, Diversity and Inclusion at Work: A Research Companion*, pp. 383–98, Cheltenham, UK and Northampton, MA: Edward Elgar.

Collyer, F. and White, K. (2011) 'The privatisation of Medicare and the National Health Service, and the global marketisation of healthcare systems', *Health Sociology Review*, 20(3): 238–44.

Colomy, P. (ed.) (1991) *Functionalist Sociology*, Hants, UK: Aldershot.

Commission on the Social Determinants of Health (CSDH) (2008) *Closing the Gap in a Generation: Health Equity Through Action on the Social Determinants of Health*, Geneva: WHO.

Connell, R. (2011) 'Steering towards equality? How gender regimes change inside the state', In R. Connell, *Confronting Equality: Gender, Knowledge and Global Change*, pp. 25–40, Sydney, Melbourne, Auckland and London: Allen & Unwin.

Connell, R. (2009) *Gender: In World Perspective*, 2nd edn, Cambridge: Polity Press.

Connell, R. (2007) *Southern Theory: The Global Dynamics of Knowledge in Social Science*, Sydney: Allen & Unwin.

Connell, R. (2002) *Gender*, Cambridge: Polity Press.

Connell, R. (1999) *Masculinities*, Berkeley and Los Angeles: Polity Press.

Connell, R. and Dados, N. (2014) 'Where in the world does neoliberalism come from? *Theory and Society*, online first DOI 10.1007/s11186-014-9212-9.

Connell, R., Fawcett, B. and Meagher, G. (2009) 'Neoliberalism, new public management and the human service professions', *Journal of Sociology*, 45(4): 331–9.

Cook, M. (2013) 'Māori smoking, alcohol and drugs: Tupeka, waipiro me te tarukino', *Te ara: The Encyclopaedia of New Zealand*, Auckland: Ministry for Culture and Heritage.

Cornelissen, S., Cheru, F. and Shaw, T.M. (eds) (2012) *African and International Relations in the 21st Century*, New York: Palgrave Macmillan.

Coser, L.A. (1971) *Masters of Sociological Thought: Ideas in Historical and Social Context*, New York, Chicago, San Francisco, Atlanta: Harcourt Brace Jovanovich.

Courtney, W. (2011) *Dying to be Men: Psychosocial, Environmental and Biobehavioral Directions in Promoting the Health of Men and Boys*, New York and London: Routledge.

Cristia, J.P. (2009) 'Rising mortality and life expectancy differentials by lifetime earnings in the United States', *Journal of Health Economics*, 2(8): 984–95.

Crow, G. (2002). *Social Solidarities: Theories, Identities and Social Change*. Buckingham: Open University Press.

Dachs, G., Currie, M., McKenzie, F., Jeffreys, M., Cox, B., Foliaki, S., Marchand, L. and Robinson, B. (2008) 'Cancer disparities in Indigenous Polynesian populations: Maori, native Hawaiians and Pacific people', *The Lancet*, 9: 473–84.

Dahlberg, F. (ed.) (1981) *Woman the Gatherer*, New Haven: Yale University Press.

Davies, J.B., Sandstrom, S., Shorrocks, A. and Wolff, E.N. (2011) 'The level and distribution of global household wealth', *The Economic Journal*, 121: 223–54.

Davison, C., Frankel, S. and Davey-Smith, G. (1992) ' "To hell with tomorrow": Coronary heart disease risk and the ethnography of fatalism', In S. Scott, G. Willliams, S. Platt and H. Thomas (eds) *Private Risks and Public Dangers*, pp. 95–111, Aldershot, Avebury.

Dean, M. (2014) 'Rethinking neoliberalism', *Journal of Sociology*, 50(2): 150–63.

DeNavas-Walt, C., Proctor, B.D. and Smith, J.C. (2011), 'Current population reports', *Income, Poverty, and Health Insurance Coverage in the United States: 2010*, pp. 60–239, Washington: US Government Printing Office.

Denton, N.A. (2006) 'Segregation and discrimination in housing', In R.G. Bratt, M.E. Stone and C. Hartman (eds) *A Right to Housing: Foundation for a New Social Agenda*, pp. 61–81, Philadelphia: Temple University Press.

Department of Prime Minister and Cabinet (2014) *Closing the Gap: Prime Minister's Report.* Accessed at: www.dpmc.gov.au, 25 April 2014.

Devaux, M. and Sassi, F. (2013) 'Social inequalities in obesity and overweight in 11 OECD countries', *European Journal of Public Health*, 23(3): 464–9.

Diamond, J.M. (2012)*The World Until Yesterday: What Can We Learn from Traditional Societies?*, New York: Viking.

Dobash, R.E. and Dobash, R.P. (2004) 'Women's violence to men in intimate relationships: Working on a puzzle', *British Journal of Criminology*, 44(3): 324–49.

Dockery, A.M. (2010) 'Culture and wellbeing: The case of Indigenous Australians', *Social Indicators Research: An International and Interdisciplinary Journal for Quality-of-Life Measurement*, 99(2): 315–32.

Dodson, M. (2004) 'Indigenous Australians', In R. Manne (ed.) *The Howard Years*, pp. 119–43, Melbourne : Black Inc. Agenda.

Dodson, M. (1997) 'Land rights and social justice', In G. Yunupiningu (ed.) *Our Land is Our Life*, pp. 39–51, Brisbane: UQP.

Dolan, K. and Kroll, L. (eds) (2013) *The Forbes 400: The Richest People in America.* Accessed at: www.forbes.com/forbes-400/, 21 June 2014.

Donner, W. and Rodriguez, H. (2008) 'Population composition, migration and inequality: The influence of demographic changes on disaster risk and vulnerability', *Social Forces*, 87(2): 1089–114.

Dorling, D. (2014) 'Thinking about class', *Sociology*, 48(3): 452–62.

Dorling, D., Mitchell, R. and Pearce, J. (2007) 'The global impact of income inequality on health by age: An observational study', *The British Medical Journal*, 335(873): 1–5. Accessed at: www. bmj.com/content/335/7625/873?tab=response-form, 19 August 2014.

Doyal, L. and Pennell, I. (1979) *The Political Economy of Health*, London: Pluto Press.

Draper, G., Turrell, G. and Oldenburg, B. (2004) *Health Inequalities in Australia: Mortality*, Health Inequalities Monitoring Series No. 1. AIHW Catalogue No. PHE 55, Canberra: Queensland University of Technology and the Australian Institute of Health and Welfare.

Drever, F. and Whitehead, M. (1997) *Health Inequalities: Decennial Supplement*, ONS, London: The Stationery Office.

Dubos, R. (1960) *Mirage of Health: Utopias, Progress and Biological Change*, London: George Allen & Unwin.

Durkheim, E. (1895/1964) *The Rules of Sociological Method* (8th edn), New York: Free Press of Glencoe.

Durkheim, E. (1893/1964) *The Division of Labor in Society*, New York: Free Press of Glencoe.

Dwyer, C. (2000) 'Negotiating diasporic identities: Young British South Asian muslim women', *Women's Studies International Forum*, 23(4): 475–86.

Dwyer, P. (2010) *Understanding Social Citizenship*, 2nd edn, Cambridge: Polity Press.

Ehrenreich, B. and English, D. (1979) *For Her Own Good: 150 Years of the Experts' Advice to Women*, London: Pluto Press.

Ehrle, L.H. and Cleveland, R.W. (2010) 'Middle class mythology and the Houdini disappearing act: Health care and jobs joined at the hip', *International Journal of Health Services*, 40(4): 667–8.

Elder, B. (2003) *Blood on the Wattle: Massacres and Maltreatment of Aboriginal Australians Since 1788*, 3rd edn, Frenchs Forest, NSW: New Holland.

Elias, N. (1994) *The Civilizing Process*, Oxford: Blackwell.

Emslie, C. and Hunt, K. (2008) 'The weaker sex? Exploring lay understandings of gender differences in life expectancy: A qualitative study', *Social Science & Medicine*, 67(5): 808–16.

Engels, F. (1844/1950) *The Condition of the Working Class in England in 1844*, London: George Allen and Unwin.

Eskes, T. and Haanen, C. (2007) 'Why do women live longer than men?' *European Journal of Obstetrics & Gynaecology and Reproductive Health*, *133*(2): 126–33.

Espinoza, H., Sequeira, M., Domingo, G., Amador, J., Quintanilla, M. and Santos, T. (2011) 'Management of the HIV epidemic in Nicaragua: The need to improve information systems and access to affordable diagnostics', *Bulletin of the World Health Organization*, DOI: 10.2471/BLT.11.086124.

Evans, R.G. (1994) 'Introduction', In R.G. Evans, M.L. Barer and T.R. Marmor (eds) *Why Are Some People Healthy and Others Not?: The Determinants of Health of Populations*, pp. 3–26, New York: Aldine de Gruyter.

Evans, R.G., Hodge, M. and Pless, I.B. (1994) 'If not genetics, then what?: Biological pathways and population health', In R.G. Evans, M.L. Barer and T.R. Marmor (eds) *Why Are Some People Healthy and Others Not?: The Determinants of Health of Populations*, pp. 161–88, New York: Aldine de Gruyter.

Everingham, C. (2003) *Social Justice and the Politics of Community*, Aldershot: Ashgate.

Fairclough, N. (1992) *Discourse and Social Change*, Cambridge: Polity Press.

Fanon, F. (1967) *Black Skin, White Masks*, New York: Grove Press.

Fanon, F. (1966) *The Wretched of the Earth*, New York: Grove Press.

Farrell, C., McAvoy, H., Wilde, J. and Combat Poverty Agency (2008) *Tackling Health Inequalities: An All-Ireland Approach to Social Determinants*, Dublin: Combat Poverty Agency/ and Institute for Public Health in Ireland.

Ferge, Z. (1997) 'The changed welfare paradigm: The individualization of the social', *Social Policy & Administration*, 31(1): 20–44.

Ferrie, J. (ed.) (2004) *Work Stress and Health: The Whitehall II Study*, London: Council of Civil Service Unions and Cabinet Office.

Figueiredo-Santos, J.A. (2011) 'Class divisions and health chances in Brazil', *International Journal of Health Services*, *41*(4): 691–708.

Fireside, D., Smriti, R., Reuss, A. and Gluckman, A. (eds) (2009) *The Wealth Inequality Reader* (3rd edn), Boston, MA: Dollars and Sense.

Fischetti; M. (2011) 'Baby's life, mother's schooling', *Scientific American*, *35*(1): 88.

Fitzpatrick, P. (2001) 'Terminal legality: Imperialism and the (de)composition of law', In D. Kirkby and C. Coleborne (eds) *Law, History and Colonialism: The Reach of Empire*, pp. 9–26, New York: Manchester University Press.

Flanagan, R. (2008) *Wanting*, Sydney: Vintage Books.

Flannery, T. (2005) *The Weathermakers: The History and Future Impact of Climate Change*, Melbourne: Text Publishing.

Food and Agriculture Organization of the United Nations (FAO) (2013) *FAO Statistical Handbook: World Food and Agriculture*, Rome: FAO.

Forbes (2013) 'The world's biggest public companies list', *Forbes*. Accessed at: www.forbes.com/global2000/list/#page:1_sort:0_direction:asc_search:_filter:Pharmaceuticals_filter:All%20countries_filter:All%20states, 26 June 2014.

Forde I., Rasanathan K. and Krech R. (2012) 'Cash transfer schemes and the health sector: Making the case for greater involvement', *Bulletin of the World Health Organization*, 90: 551–3.

Fortune Magazine (2013) 'Global 500'. Accessed at: http://money.cnn.com/magazines/fortune/global500/2013/full_list/, 25 February 2014.

Foucault, M. (1980) *Power/Knowledge: Selected Interviews and Other Writings 1972–1977*, edited by Colin Gordon, New York: Harvester Wheatsheaf.

Foucault, M. (1976) *The Birth of the Clinic: An Archaeology of Medical Perception*, London: Tavistock.

Fraser, N. (1989) *Unruly Practices: Power, Discourse and Gender in Contemporary Social Theory*, Cambridge: Polity Press.

Fredrickson, G. (2002) *Racism: A Short History*, Princeton: Princeton University Press.

Freidson, E. (1970) *Professional Dominance: The Social Structure of Medical Care*, New Brunswick, US: Traction.

Friedman, T.L. (2006) *The World is Flat: A Brief History of the Twenty-First Century*, Camberwell, Vic.: Penguin.

Fuchs, D.A. (2007) *Business Power in Global Governance*, Boulder, CO: Lynne Rienner Publishers.

Fukuyama, F. (2011) *The Origins of Political Order*, New York: Farrar, Straus and Giroux.

Garnett, S. and Sithole, B. (2007) *Sustainable Northern Landscapes and the Nexus with Indigenous Health: Healthy Country, Healthy People*, Canberra: Land and Water Australia.

Geggus, D. (2012) 'Rights, resistance and emancipation: A response to Robin Blackburn', In K.E. Tunstall (ed.) *Self-Evident Truths?: Human Rights and the Enlightenment*, pp. 157–67, New York and London: Bloomsbury.

Geras, N. and Wokler, R. (eds) (2000) *The Enlightenment and Modernity*, New York: St Martin's Press.

Giddens, A. (2012) *The Consequences of Modernity*, Oxford: Wiley.

Giddens, A. (2009) *Sociology*, Cambridge: Polity Press.

Giddens, A. and Sutton, P.W. (2014) *Essential Concepts in Sociology*, Cambridge: Polity Press.

Gideon, J. (2013) 'Migrant health and illhealth in Johannesburg: Migration and inequality', In T. Bastia (ed.) *Migration and Inequality*, pp. 121–44, London: Abingdon.

Gil, A. and Vega, W. (2010) 'Alcohol, tobacco and other drugs', In M. Aguirre-Molina, L.N. Borrell and W. Vega (eds) *Health Issues in Latino Males: A Social and Structural Approach*, pp. 99–122, New Brunswick, New Jersey and London: Rutgers University Press.

Gilbert, J. (2007) 'Historical Indigenous peoples' land claims: A comparative and international approach to the common law doctrine on Indigenous title', *International and Comparative Law Quarterly*, 56: 583–612.

Gilbert, L. and Selikow, T.A. (2012) 'HIV/AIDS and gender', In E. Kuhlmann and E. Annandale (eds) 2nd edn *The Palgrave Handbook of Gender and Healthcare*, pp. 209–23, Houndmills, Basingstoke: Palgrave Macmillan.

Gilman, S.L. (2010) *Obesity: The Biography*, Oxford: Oxford University Press.

Gilman, S.L. (2000) *Making the Body Beautiful: A Cultural History of Aesthetic Surgery*, Oxford: Oxford University Press.

Gilroy, J., Donelly, M., Colmar, S. and Parmenter, T. (2013) 'Conceptual framework for policy and research development with Indigenous people with disabilities', *Australian Aboriginal Studies: Journal of the Australian Institute of Aboriginal and Torres Strait Islander Studies*, 2: 42–57.

Gilson, L., Doherty, J., Loewenson, R. and Francis, V. (2007) *Final Report of World Health Organization Knowledge Network on Health Systems of the World Health Organization Commission on the Social Determinants of Health*, London: Centre for Health Policy at the University of the Witwatersrand, South Africa, EQUINET and the Health Policy Unit of the London School of Hygiene and Tropical Medicine.

Ginter, E. and Simko, V. (2013) 'Women live longer than men', *Britislava Medical Journal*, 114(2): 45–9.

Gleeson, L. (1993) *Love Me, Love Me Not*, Melbourne: Penguin.

Gleeson, T. (2014) *Middle Managers: Evaluating Australia's Biggest Management Resource*, Melbourne: Australian Institute of Management. Accessed at: http://www.aim.com.au/research/default.html, 4 September 2014.

Graham, H., Inskip, H.M., Francis, B. and Harman, J. (2006) 'Pathways of disadvantage and smoking careers: Evidence and policy implications', *Journal of Epidemiology and Community Health*, 60(Suppl.): ii7–12.

Grossman, C.L. (2012) 'Number of US mosques up 75% since 2000', *USA Today*, 29 February, Accessed at: http://usatoday30.usatoday.com/news/religion/story/2012-02-29/islamic-worship-growth-us/53298792/1, 7 February 2014.

Guile, M. (2011) *Charlie Perkins and the Freedom Ride*, South Yarra: Macmillan.

Gupta, S., Verhoven, M. and Tiongson, E.R. (2003) 'Public spending on health care and the poor', *Health Economics*, 12(8): 685–96.

Gushulak, B.D., Pottie, K., Hatcher-Roberts, J., Torres, S. and DesMeules, M. (2011) 'Migration and health in Canada: Health in the global village', *Canadian Medical Association Journal*, 183(12): E952–8

Haddad, S., Mohindra, K., Siekmans, K., Mak, G. and Narayana, D. (2012) 'Health divide between indigenous and non-indigenous populations in Kerala, India: Population based study', *BMC Public Health*, 12.

Hall, C. (2013) *White, Male and Middle Class: Explorations in Feminism and History*, Hobokin: John Wiley & Sons.

Hall, C. (2002) *Civilising Subjects: Metropole and Colony in the English Imagination, 1830–1867*, Chicago: University of Chicago Press.

Hall, S. (1997) 'The work of representation', In S. Hall, *Representations: Cultural Representations and Signifying Practices*, pp. 15–64, London: Sage, in association with The Open University.

Hamalainen, P., Saarela, K. and Takala, J. (2009) 'Global trend according to estimated number of occupational accidents and fatal work-related diseases to region and country level', *Journal of Safety Reseach*, 40: 125–39.

Hancock, D. (1995) *Citizens of the World: London Merchants and the Integration of the British Atlantic Community*, Cambridge, New York and Melbourne: Cambridge University Press.

Hardy-Fanta, C. (2006) *Intersectionality and Politics: Recent Research on Gender, Race, and Political Representation in the United States*, New York: Haworth Press.

Harley, K., Willis, K., Gabe, J., Short, S., Collyer, F., Natalier, K. and Calnan, M. (2011) 'Constructing health consumers: Private health insurance discourses in Australia and the United Kingdom', *Health Sociology Review*, 20(3): 306–20.

Hartman, C.W. and Squires G.D. (eds) (2007) *There is No Such Thing as a Natural Disaster: Race, Class and Hurricane Katrina*, New York: Routledge.

Harvey, D. (2010) *The Enigma of Capital and the Crises of Capitalism*, Oxford and New York: Oxford University Press.

Harvey, D. (2005) *A Brief History of Neoliberalism*, Oxford: Oxford University Press.

Havnevik, K. (1987) *The IMF and the World Bank in Africa: Conditionality, Impact and Alternatives*, Uppsala: Nordiska Afrikainstitute.

Health Canada (2009) *A Statistical Profile on the Health of First Nations in Canada: Self-rated Health and Selected Conditions, 2002 to 2005*, Ottowa: Health Canada. Accessed at: www.hc-sc.gc.ca/fniah-spnia/pubs/aborig-autoch/index-eng.php, 25 April 2014.

Health Canada (2006) *Healthy Canadians: A Federal Report on Comparable Health Indicators 2006*, Ottowa: Health Canada. Accessed at: www.hc-sc.gc.ca/hcs-sss/pubs/system-regime/index-eng.php, 25 April 2014.

Healy, J. and Dugdale, P. (2013) *The Australian HealthCare System*, Canberra: Australian National University.

Hellander, I. (2011) 'The deepening crisis in US health care: A review of data', *International Journal of Health Services*, 41(3): 575–86.

Henderson, S. and Petersen, A. (2001) *Consuming Health: The Commodification of Health Care*, London: Routledge.

Hennekens, C. and Buring, J. (1987) *Epidemiology in Medicine*, Boston, MA: Little, Brown and Co.

Hill, C. (1972) *The World Turned Upside Down: Radical Ideas During the English Revolution*, London: Temple Smith.

Hill, C. (1969) *Reformation to Industrial Revolution, 1530–1780*, Harmondsworth: Penguin.

Hill, L. (2007) *Someone Knows My Name*, London, New York, Sydney and Auckland: Fourth Estate – Harper Collins.

Himmelstein, D.U., Thorne, D., Warren, E. and Woolhandler, S. (2009) 'Medical bankruptcy in the United States, 2007: Results of a national study', *The American Journal of Medicine*, 122(8): 741–6.

Ho, C. and Alcorso, C. (2004) 'Migrants and employment: Challenging the success story', *Journal of Sociology*, 40(3): 237–59.

Hobsbawm, E. (1994) *The Age of Extremes: The Short Twentieth Century, 1914–1991*, London: Abacus.

Hobsbawm, E. (1992) *Nations and Nationalism Since 1780: Programme, Myth, Reality*, Cambridge: Cambridge University Press.

Hobsbawm, E. (1987) *The Age of Empire 1875–1914*, London: Abacus.

Hobsbawm, E. (1969a) *Industry and Empire: From 1750 to Present Day*, London: Penguin.

Hobsbawm, E. (1969b) 'Introduction', In F. Engels (ed.) *The Condition of the Working Class in England*, pp. 7–17, London: Panther.

Hodgson, H. (2014) 'The super rich and tax: Lifters or leaners?' *The Conversation*. Accessed at: https://theconversation.com/the-super-rich-and-tax-lifters-or-leaners-27700, 13 June 2014.

Holden, R.H. and Villars, R. (2013) *Contemporary Latin America: 1970 to the Present*, Oxford: Blackwell.

Hollingsworth, B. (2008) 'The measurement of efficiency and productivity of health care delivery', *Health Economics*, 17(10): 1107–28.

Homedes, N. and Ugalde, A. (2005) 'Why neoliberal health reforms have failed in Latin America', *Health Policy*, 71(1): 83–96.

Honneth, A. (2007) *Disrespect: The Normative Foundations of Critical Theory*, Cambridge: Polity Press.

Honneth, A. (1995) *The Struggle for Recognition: The Moral Grammar of Social Conflicts*, Cambridge, MA: Polity Press.

House of Representatives Standing Committee on Aboriginal Affairs (1987) *Return to Country: The Aboriginal Homelands Movement in Australia*, Canberra: Australian Government Printing Service.

Houweling, T.A.J., Kunst, A.E., Looman, C.W.N & Mackenbach, J.P. (2005) 'Determinants of under-5 mortality among the poor and the rich: A cross-national analysis of 43 developing countries', *International Journal of Epidemiology*, 34(6): 1257–65.

Huffpost Celebrity (2013) 'Kim Kardashian's baby: All is well after major pregnancy scare', *Huffington Post*, 17 June. Accessed at: www.huffingtonpost.com/2013/o6/17/kim-kardashian-baby-health-scare_n_3453181.html, 28 August 2014.

Humphrey, C. (2004) 'Place, space and reputation: The changing role of Harley Street in English healthcare', *Journal of Social Theory and Health*, 2(2): 153–69.

Hunter, E. (1993) *Aboriginal Health and History: Power and Prejudice in Remote Australia*, New York: Cambridge University Press.

Husain, F. and O'Brien, M. (2000) 'Muslim communities in Europe: Reconstruction and transformation', *Current Sociology*, 48(4): 1–13.

Hyde, J.S. (2005) 'The gender similarities hypothesis', *American Psychologist*, 60(6): 581–92.

Intergovernmental Panel on Climate Change (IPCC) (2014) *Climate Change 2014: Impacts, Adaptation, and Vulnerability*. Accessed at: www.ipcc.ch/report/ar5/wg2/, 23 June 2013.

International Labor Office (ILO) (2014) 'Occupational safety and health profile: Bangla Desh', *Country Profiles on Occupational Safety and Health*. Accessed at: www.ilo.org/safework/countries/asia/bangladesh/lang–en/index.htm, 5 September 2014.

ILO (2013) *Promotional Framework For Occupational Safety and Health*. Accessed at: www.ilo.org/wcmsp5/groups/public/@ed_protect/@protrav/@safework/documents/meetingdocument/wcms_111296.pdf, 23 June 2014.

International Organization for Migration (IOM) (2014) *Costa Rica*, Geneva: IOM. Accessed at: www.iom.int/cms/en/sites/iom/home/where-we-work/americas/central-and-north-america-and-th/costa-rica.html, 28 August 2014.

IOM (2013) *International Migration, Health and Human Rights*, Geneva: IOM.

Jaworski, K. (2014) *The Gender of Suicide: Knowledge Production, Theory and Suicidology*, Surrey, UK: Ashgate.

Johnson, T. (1995) Governmentality and the institutionalisation of expertise, In T. Johnson (ed.) *Health Professions and the State in Europe*, pp. 7–24, London: Routledge.

Kabeer, N. (2006) 'Poverty, social exclusion and the MDGs: The challenge of "durable inequalities" in the Asian context', *IDS Bulletin*, 37(3): 64–78.

Kawachi, I., Daniels, N. and Robinson, D.E. (2005) 'Health disparities by race and class: Why both matter', *Health Affairs*, 24(2): 343–52.

Kelly, J.E. (ed.) (2002) *Industrial Relations: Labour Markets, Labour Process and Trade Unionism*, London: Routledge.

Kelly, K., Dudgeon, P., Gee, G. and Glaskin, B. (2010) *Living on the Edge: Social and Emotional Wellbeing and Risk and Protective Factors for Serious Psychological Distress Among Aboriginal and Torres Strait Islander People*, Discussion Paper No. 10, Darwin: Cooperative Research Centre for Aboriginal Health.

Kendig, H. (2004) 'The social sciences and successful aging: Issues for Asia–Oceania', *Geriatrics & Gerontology International*, 4: S6–11.

Kendig, H. and Browning, C. (2010). 'A social view on healthy ageing: Multi-disciplinary perspectives and Australian evidence', In D. Dannefer and C. Phillipson (eds), *The Sage Handbook of Social Gerontology*, pp. 459–471, Thousand Oaks: Sage.

Kendig, H. and Phillipson, C. (2014) 'Building age-friendly communities: New approaches to challenging health and social inequalities', In The British Academy (ed.) *If You Could Do One Thing: Nine Local Actions to Reduce Health Inequalities*, pp. 102–11, London: The British Academy.

Kennedy, S. and McDonald, J.T. (2006) 'Immigrant health in the period after arrival in Australia', In D.A. Cobb-Clark and S. Khoo (eds) *Public Policy and Immigrant Settlement*, pp. 149–74, Cheltenham, Vic.: Elgar Publishing.

Kenny, D.T. (2013) *Bringing Up Baby: The Psychoanalytic Infant Comes of Age*, London: Karnac.

Kida, T.M. and Mackintosh, M. (2005) 'Public expenditure allocation and incidence under health care market liberalization: A Tanzanian case study', In M. Mackintosh and M. Koivusalo (eds) *Commercialization of Health Care: Global and Local Dynamics and Policy Responses*. Basingstoke: Palgrave Macmillan.

Kidd, R. (2006) *Trustees on Trial: Recovering the Stolen Wages*, Canberra: Aboriginal Studies Press.

Kochanek, K., Xu, J., Murphy, S. and Minino, A. (2011) 'Deaths: Final data for 2009', *National Vital Statistics Reports*, 60(3): 1–117. Accessed at: www.cdc.gov/nchs, 1 April 2014.

Kolb, B. and Gibb, R. (2011) 'Brain plasticity and behaviour in the developing brain', *Journal of Canadian Academy of Child and Adolescent Psychiatry*, 20(4): 265–76.

Kondilis, E., Giannakopoulos, S., Gavana, M., Ierodiakonou, I., Waitzkin, H. and Benos, A. (2013) 'Economic crisis, restrictive policies, and the population's health and health care: The Greek case', *American Journal of Public Health*, e1–e8. Accessed at: www.phmovement.org/ sites/www.phmovement.org/files/Kondilis%20et%20al%20(2013)%20Economic%20crisis%20 restrictive%20policies%20and%20health%20Greece%20(1).pdf.

Kuhlmann, E. and Annandale, E. (2012) 'Researching transformations in health services and policy in international perspective: An introduction', *Current Sociology*, 60(4): 401–14.

Kulkarni, S.C., Levin-Rector, A., Ezzati, M. and Murray, C.J.L. (2011) 'Falling behind: Life expectancy in US counties from 2000 to 2007 in an international context', *Population Health Metrics*, 9: 16, 15 June.

Kumar, U.A. (2013) 'India has just one doctor for every 1,700 people', *The New Indian Express*, 22 September. Accessed at: www.newindianexpress.com/magazine/India-has-just-one-doctor-for-every-1700-people/2013/09/22/article1792010.ece#.UvlpTGKSyQw, 11 February 2014.

Labonte, R. and Laverack, G. (2001) 'Capacity building in health promotion; Part 1: For whom? And for what purpose?', *Critical Public Health*, 11(2): 111–27.

LaGarde M. and Palmer, N. (2006) 'The impact of health financing strategies on access to health services in low and middle income countries: Protocol', *Cochrane Database of Systematic Reviews*, Issue 3, Art. No: CD006092. doi: 10.1002/14651858.CD006092.

Lahelma, E., Martikainen, P., Laaksonen, M. and Aittomaki, A. (2004) 'Pathways between socioeconomic determinants of health', *Journal of Epidemiology and Community Health*, 58: 327–32.

Lang, J., Greig, A. and Connell, R. (2008) *Women 2000 and Beyond: The Role of Men and Boys in Achieving Gender Equality*, New York: United Nations Division for the Advancement of Women, Department of Economic and Social Affairs.

Langlois, K., Findlay, L. and Kohen, D. (2013) 'Dietary habits of Aboriginal children', *Statistics Canada Health Reports*, Catalogue No. 82–003-x. Accessed at: www.statcan.gc.ca, 1 April 2014.

Lao Ministry of Health (2011) *Ethnic Group Development Plan*, Catalogue No. IPP495. Accessed at: www.worldbank.org, 1 May 2014.

Larkin, G. (1983) *Occupational Monopoly and Modern Medicine*, London: Tavistock.

Last, J. (ed.) (2001) *A Dictionary of Epidemiology*, New York: Oxford University Press.

Laverack, G. (2006) 'Improving health outcomes through community empowerment: A review of the literature', *Journal of Health Population and Nutrition*, 24(1): 113–20.

Lee, K., McGuinness, C. and Kawakami, T. (2011) *Research on Occupational Safety and Health for Migrant Workers in Five Asian Pacific Countries: Australia, Republic of Korea, Malaysia, Singapore and Thailand*, ILO Asia and the Pacific Working Paper Series, ILO.

Lehndorff, S. (2012) 'The triumph of failed ideas: Introduction', In S. Lehndorff (ed.) *A Triumph of Failed Ideas: European Models of Capitalism in Crisis*, pp. 7–26, Brussels: The European Trade Union Institute.

Lewis, J.M. (2005) *Health Policy and Politics: Networks, Ideas and Power*, Melbourne: IP Communications.

Lewis, K., Burd-Sharps, S. and Sachs, J. (2010) *The Measure of America, 2010–2011: Mapping Risks and Resilience*, New York: NYU Press.

Lindsay, J.M. (2006) 'A big night out in Melbourne: Drinking as an enactment of class and gender', *Contemporary Drug Problems: An Interdisciplinary Quarterly*, 33(1): 29–61.

Lisk, F., Besada, H. and Martin, P. (2013) *Regulating Extraction in the Global South: Towards a Framework for Accountability*, Background Research Paper, UN High Level Panel on the Post-2015 Development Agenda. Accessed at: www.post2015hlp.org/wp-content/uploads/2013/06/Lisk-Besada-Martin_Regulating-Extraction-in-the-Global-South-Towards-a-Framework-for-Accountability-_FINALFINAL.pdf, 5 September 2014.

Lister, J. (2007) *Globalisation and Health Systems Change*, Ottawa: World Health Organization Commission on Social Determinants of Health Globalization and Health Knowledge Network and Institute of Population Health Globalisation and Health Equity.

Locke, J. (1690/1948) *Second Treatise of Civil Government and a Letter Concerning Toleration*, edited by J.W. Gough, Oxford: Basil Blackwell.

Long, D., Forsyth, R., Iedema, R. and Carroll, K. (2006) 'The (im)possibilities of clinical democracy', *Health Sociology Review*, 15(5): 106–19.

Lopez, A.D., Mathers, C.D., Ezzati, M., Jamison, D.Y. and Murray, C.J.L. (2006) 'Global and regional burden of disease and risk factors, 2001: Systematic analysis of population health data', *Lancet*, 367(9524): 1747–57.

Lovejoy, P.E. (1989) 'The impact of the Atlantic slave trade on Africa: A review of the literature', *Journal of African History*, 30(3): 365–94.

Loxley, W, Gray, D., Wilkinson, C., Chikritzhs, T., Midford, R. and Moore, D. (2005) 'Alcohol policy and harm reduction in Australia', *Drug and Alcohol Review*, 24(6): 559–68.

Luis R.L. (2013) 'Cuba: External debt and finance in the context of limited reforms', In *Cuba in Transition Volume 23 Papers and Proceedings of the Twenty-Third Annual Meeting of the Association for the Study of the Cuban Economy* (ASCE), pp. 186–94, Florida, Miami: ASCE.

Luiten van Zanden, J., Buringh, E. and Bosker, M. (2010) *The Rise and Decline of European Parliaments 1188–1789*, Discussion Paper No. 7809, London: Centre for Economic Policy Research. Accessed at: http://vkc.library.uu.nl/vkc/seh/research/Lists/Research%20Desk/Attachments/14/the%20rise%20and%20decline%20of%20european%20parliaments.pdf, 5 September 2014.

Lukes, S. (2005) *Power: A Radical View,* 2nd edn, New York: Palgrave Macmillan.

Lukes, S. (1973) *Individualism: Key Concepts in the Social Sciences*, Oxford: Basil Blackwell.

Macdonald, K.M. (1995) *The Sociology of the Professions*, London: Sage.

MacDorman, M., Kirmeyer, S. and Wilson, E. (2012) 'Fetal and perinatal mortality, United States, 2006', *National Vital Statistics Report*, 60(8): 1–23. Accessed at: www.cdc.gov/nchs, 1 April 2014.

MacFarlane, A. (1978) *The Origins of English Individualism*, Oxford: Basil Blackwell.

Mackintosh, M. and Koivusalo, M. (eds) (2005) *Commercialization of health care: Global and local dynamics and policy responses. Social Policy in a Development Context*. Basingstoke, UK: Palgrave Macmillan.

Magdoff, F. and Tokar, B. (2010) 'Agriculture and food in crisis: An overview', In F. Magdoff and B. Tokar (eds) *Agriculture and Food in Crisis: Conflict, Resistance and Renewal*, pp. 9–30, New York: Monthly Review Press.

Malqvist, M., Hoa, D.T.P., Liem, N.T., Thorson, A. and Thomsen, S. (2013) 'Ethnic minority health in Vietnam: A review exposing horizontal inequity', *Global Health Action*, 6: 1–19.

Marmot, M. (2006) 'Introduction', In M. Marmot and R.G. Wilkinson (eds) *Social Determinants of Health*, 2nd edn, pp. 1–5, Oxford: Oxford University Press.

Marmot, M., Allen, J., Bell, R., Bloomer, E. and Goldblatt, P. (2012) 'WHO European review of social determinants of health and the health divide', *Lancet*, 380(9846): 1011–29.

Marmot, M. and Shipley, M.J. (1996) 'Do socioeconomic differences in health persist after retirement? 25 year follow up of civil servants from the first Whitehall study', *The British Medical Journal*, 313: 1177–80.

Marmot, M. and Wilkinson, R.G. (eds) (2006) *Social Determinants of Health*, 2nd edn, Oxford: Oxford University Press.

Martin, A.B., Hartman, M., Whittle, L., Catlin, A. and the National Health Expenditures Account Team (2014) 'National health spending in 2012: Rate of health spending growth remained low for the fourth consecutive year', *Health Affairs*, 33(1): 67–77.

Marx, K. (1852/1963) *The Eighteenth Brumaire of Louis Bonaparte: With Explanatory Notes*, New York: International Publishers.

Marx, K. (1845/1969) Theses on Feuerbach, In L.S. Feuer (ed.) *Marx and Engels: Basic Writings on Politics and Philosophy*, London and Glasgow: Collins/Fontana.

Massey, D.S. and Denton, N.A. (1993) *American Apartheid: Segregation and the Making of the Underclass*, Harvard: Harvard University Press.

Massola, J. (2014) 'Tony Abbott's war on red tape starts with repeal day', *Sydney Morning Herald*, 17 March.

Mayhew, H. (1861) *London Labour and the London Poor*. Accessed at: www.etext.virginia.edu/toc/modeng/public/MayLond.html, 17 June 2013.

McAllister, T.W. and Stein, M.B. (2010) 'Effects of psychological and biomechanical trauma on brain and behavior', *Annals of the New York Academy of Sciences*, 1208: 46–57.

McEwen, B.S. (2008) 'Central effects of stress hormones in health and disease: Understanding the protective and damaging effects of stress and stress mediators', *European Journal of Pharmacology*, 583(1–2): 174–85.

McKeown, T., Record, R.G. and Turner, R.D. (1975) 'An interpretation of the decline of mortality in England and Wales in the twentieth century', *Population Studies*, 29: 391–422.

McKinlay, J.B. and McKinlay, S.M. (2009) 'Medical measures and the decline of mortality', In P. Conrad (ed.) *The Sociology of Health and Illness: Critical Perspectives*, 8th edn, New York: Worth Publishers.

McKinlay, J.B. and Stoeckle, J.D. (1988) 'Corporatization and the social transformation of doctoring', *International Journal of Health Services*, 18(2): 191–205.

McLennan, V. and Khavarpour, F. (2004) 'Culturally appropriate health promotion: Its meaning and application in Aboriginal communities', *Health Promotion Journal of Australia*, 15(3): 37–9.

McMichael, P. (2010) 'The world food crisis in historical perspective', In F. Magdoff and B. Tokar (eds) *Agriculture and Food in Crisis: Conflict, Resistance and Renewal*, pp. 33–50, New York: Monthly Review Press.

McMichael, A., Friel, S., Nyong, A. and Corvalan, C. (2008) 'Global environmental change and health: Impacts, inequalities, and the health sector', *British Medical Journal*, 336(7637): 191–4.

McNeilage, A. (2013) 'Islamic student numbers soar', *The Sydney Morning Herald*, 4 August. Accessed at: www.smh.com.au/nsw/islamic-student-numbers-soar-20130803-2r668.html, 4 September 2014.

Meagher, G. and Szebehely, M. (eds) (2013) *Marketisation in Nordic Eldercare: A Research Report on Legislation, Oversight, Extent and Consequences*, Stockholm Studies in Social Work 30, Stockholm: Department of Social Work, Stockholm University.

Medicare News Group (2014) 'What is the American Medical Association's position on the Affordable Care Act?' Accessed at: www.medicarenewsgroup.com/news/medicare-faqs/individual-faq?faqId=d7a04b02–28b7–47dd-a838–88561f629624, 23 March 2014.

Meekosha, H. (2011) 'Decolonising disability: Thinking and acting globally', *Disability and Society*, 26(6): 667–82.

Menacker, F. and Hamilton, B.E. (2010) 'Recent trends in cesarean delivery in the United States', *NCHS Data Brief, No. 35*, Hyattsville, MD: National Center for Health Statistics.

Mesa-Lago, C. (2007) 'Social security in Latin America: Pension and health care reforms in the last quarter century', *Latin American Research Review*, 42(2): 181–201.

Mill, J.S. (1910/1972) *Utilitarianism, On Liberty, and Considerations on Representative Government*, London: J.M. Dent & Sons.

Mitra, S.K. (2005) *The Puzzle of India's Governance: Culture, Context and Comparative Theory*, Milton Park: Routledge.

Modood, T. (1990) 'British Asian Muslims and the Rushdie affair', In J. Donald and A. Rattansi (eds) *'Race', Culture and Difference*, London: Sage.

Mohummadally, A. (2014) 'Growing up different in Australia', *ABC Radio National*, The Drawing Room, 10 February 2014. Accessed at: www.abc.net.au/radionational/programs/drawingroom/growing-up-muslim-in-australia/5250400, 11 February 2014.

Montagu, A. (1972) *Statement on Race*, 3rd edn, London: Oxford University Press.

Montenegro, R. and Stephens, C. (2006) 'Indigenous health in Latin America and the Caribbean: Indigenous health 2', *The Lancet*, 367(3): 1859–69.

Moore, M. (1996) *Women in the Mines: Stories of Life and Work*, New York: Twayne Publishers.

Moran, M. (2002) 'Review article: Understanding the regulatory state', *British Journal of Political Science*, 32(2): 391–413.

Moretti, E. (2012) *The New Geography of Jobs*, Boston and New York: Houghton Mifflin Harcourt.

Morrell, R. (2001) *Changing Men in South Africa*, London: University of Natal Press, Zed Books.

Mourdoukoutas, P. (2013) 'World's 500 Largest Companies in 2013: The Chinese are Rising, *Forbes*. Accessed at www.forbes.com, 25 February 2014.

Muldoon, K.A., Galway, L.P., Nakajima, M., Kanters, S., Hogg, R.S., Bendavid, E. and Mills, E.J. (2011) 'Health systems determinants of infant child and maternal mortality: A cross-sectional study of UN member countries', *Globalization and Health*, 7: 42. Accessed at: www.globalizationandhealth.com/content/7/1/42, 8 September 2014.

Munoz, N.S. and Scrimshaw, C. (1995) *The Nutrition and Health Transition of Democratic Costa Rica*, Boston, MA: International Fund for Developing Countries.

Murray, C., Kulkarni, S.C., Michaud, C., Tomijima, N., Bulzacchelli, M.T., Iandiorio, T.J., Ezzati, M. (2006) 'Eight Americas: Investigating mortality disparities across races, counties, and race-counties in the United States', *PLoS Medicine*, 3(9): e260.

Nazroo, J.Y. (2014) 'Ethnic inequalities in health: Addressing a significant gap in current evidence and policy', In The British Academy (ed.) *'If You Could Do One Thing': Nine Local Actions to Reduce Health Inequalities*, pp. 91–101, London: The British Academy.

Nazroo, J.Y. and Williams, D.R. (2006) 'The social determination of ethnic/racial inequalities in health', In Marmot, M. and Wilkinson, R.G. (eds) *Social Determinants of Health*, 2nd edn, pp. 238–66, Oxford: Oxford University Press.

New Zealand Ministry of Health (2013) *Fetal and Infant Deaths 2010*, Wellington: Ministry of Health.

New Zealand Ministry of Health (2012) *The Health of New Zealand Adults 2011/12: Key Findings of the New Zealand Health Survey*, Wellington: Ministry of Health.

New Zealand Ministry of Health (2010) *Tatau Kahukura: Maori Health Chart Book*, 2nd edn, Wellington: Ministry of Health.

Ng, F. and Aksoy, M.A. (2008) *Who Are the Net Food Importing Countries?*, Policy Research Working Paper 4457, Washington, DC: World Bank. Accessed at: https://openknowledge.worldbank.org/handle/10986/6454.

Northern Territory Department of Primary Industries, Fisheries and Mines (2008) *Annual Report 2007–08*. Accessed at: www.nt.gov.au/d/publications/, 7 May 2014.

Norton, M.I. and Ariely, D. (2011) 'Building a better America – one wealth quintile at a time, *Perspectives on Psychological Science*, 6(1): 9–12.

Norwitz, E.R. (2014) 'Prevention of spontaneous, preterm birth', *UptoDate*. Accessed at: www. uptodate.com/contents/prevention-of-spontaneous-preterm-birth, 5 September 2014.

O'Brien, R. and Elder, C. (2013) 'New ways for exploring who knows what in a native title case: A sociological approach', *Australian Aboriginal Studies: Journal of the Australian Institute of Aboriginal and Torres Strait Islander Studies*, 2: 29–41.

O'Connor, J., Orloff, A. and Shaver, S. (1999) *States, Markets, Families: Gender, Liberalism and Social Policy in Australia, Canada, Great Britain and the United States*, Cambridge: Cambridge University Press.

O'Donnell, O., van Doorslaer, E., Rannan-Eliya, R., Somanathan, A., Adhikiri, S., Harbianto, D., et al. Garg, C.C., Hanvoravongchai, P., Huq, M.N., Karan, A., Leung, G.M., Ng, C.W., Pande, B.R., Tin, K., Tisayaticom, K., Trisnantoro, L., Zhang, Y. and Zhao Y. (2007) 'The incidence of public spending on healthcare: Comparative evidence from Asia', *The World Bank Economic Review*, 21(1): 93–123. Accessed at: http://wber.oxfordjournals.org/content/21/1/93.short, 14 January 2014.

Offe, C. (1996) *Modernity and the State*, Cambridge: Polity Press.

Ohenjo, N., Willis, R., Jackson, D., Nettleton, C., Good, K. and Mugarura, B. (2006) 'Health of Indigenous people in Africa: Indigenous health 3', *Lancet*, 367: 1937–46.

Oliver, D. and Buchanan, J. (2014) 'Australian business gets a good deal from the minimum wage', *The Conversation*. Accessed at: https://theconversation.com/australian-business-gets-a-good-deal-from-the-minimum-wage-27698, 13 June 2014.

Oliver, L., Peters, P. and Kohen, D. (2012) 'Mortality rates among children and teenagers living in Inuit Nunangat 1994 to 2008', *Statistics Canada Health Report*, 23(3) Catalogue No. 82–003-X.

Oliver, M. (1996) *Understanding Disability, From Theory to Practice*, London: Macmillan.

Olshansky, S.J., Antonucci, T., Berkman, L., Binstock, R.H., Boersch-Supan, A., Cacioppo, J.T., Carnes, B.A., Carstensen, L.L., Fried, L.P., Goldman, D.P., Jackson, J., Kohli, M., Rother, J., Zheng, Y. and Rowe, J. (2012) 'Differences in life expectancy due to race and educational differences are widening, and many may not catch up', *Health Affairs*, 31(8): 1803–13.

Organization for Economic Co-operation and Development (OECD) (2013a) 'Doctors', *OECD Factbook 2013: Economic, Environmental and Social Statistics*. Accessed at: http://dx.doi.org/10.1787/factbook-2013-en, 5 September 2014.

OECD (2013b) *Health at a Glance 2013: OECD Indicators*. Accessed at: www.oecd.org/els/health-systems/Health-at-a-Glance-2013.pdf, 23 June 2014.

OECD (2013c) 'Health expenditure', *OECD Factbook 2013: Economic, Environmental and Social Statistics*. Accessed at: http://dx.doi.org/10.1787/factbook-2013-en, 5 September 2014.

OECD (2013d) 'Total tax revenue', *OECD Factbook 2013: Economic, Environmental and Social Statistics*. Accessed at: http://dx.doi.org/10.1787/factbook-2013-en, 5 September 2014.

OECD (2011a) *Consumption Tax Trends 2010: VAT/GST and Excise Rates, Trends and Administration Issues*. Accessed at: www.oecd-ilibrary.org/taxation/consumption-tax-trends-2010_ctt-2010-en, 23 June 2014.

OECD (2011b) *Help Wanted? Providing and Paying for Long-Term Care*, OECD. Accessed at: www.oecd.org/els/health-systems/helpwantedprovidingandpayingforlong-termcare.htm, 27 June 2014.

Ottersen, O.P., Dasgupta, J., Blouin, C., Buss, P., Chongsuviatwong, J.F., Frenk, J. and Scheel, I.B. (2014) 'The political origins of health inequity: Prospects for change', *The Lancet*, 33(9917): 630–67.

Oxford English Dictionary (1964) *The Concise Oxford Dictionary of Current English*, 5th edn, London: Oxford University Press.

Pahl, R.E. (1984) *Divisions of Labour*, Oxford: Basil Blackwell.

Palmer, G. and Short, S.D. (2014) *Health Care and Public Policy: An Australian Analysis*, 5th edn, Melbourne: Palgrave Macmillan.

Palmer, N., Mueller, D., Gilson, L., Mills, A., and Haines, A. (2004) 'Health financing to promote access in low income settings: How much do we know?' *Lancet*, 364: 1365–70.

Parkin, M., Sitas, F., Chirenje, M., Stein, L., Abratt, R. and Wabinga, H. (2008) 'Part 1: Cancer in Indigenous Africans – Burden, distribution, and trends', *Lancet*, 9: 683–92.

Penrose, J. and Mole, R. (2008) 'Nation-states and national identity', In K. Cox, M. Low, and J. Robinson (eds) *The SAGE Handbook of Political Geography*, pp. 271–85, London: Sage.

People's Health Movement, Medact, Health Action International, Medicos International and Third World Network (2011) *Global Health Watch: An Alternative World Health Report*, London: Zed Books.

Phillips, A. (1995) *The Politics of Presence*, Oxford: Clarendon Press.

Pickard, S. (2010) 'The role of governmentality in the establishment, maintenance and demise of professional jurisdictions: the case of geriatric medicine', *Sociology of Health & Illness*, 32(7): 1072–86.

Pilat, D., Cimper, A., Olsen, K. and Webb, C. (2006) *The Changing Nature of Manufacturing in OECD Economies*, OECD Directorate for Science, Technology and Industry Working Paper 2006/9. Accessed at: www.oecd/sti/working-papers, 27 February 2014.

Pini, B. and Mayes, R. (2008) 'Women and mining in contemporary Australia: An exploratory study', *Proceedings of the Annual Conference of the Australian Sociological Association, Melbourne, 2008*. Accessed at: www.tasa.org.au/conferences/conferencepapers08/rural.html, 2 September 2014.

Plies, J., Lucas, J. and Ward, B. (2009) *Summary of Health Statistics for US Adults: National Health Interview Survey 2008*, National Centre for Health Statistics, 10, 242, Congress Catalogue No. 362.1'0973'021s-dc21.

Pollock, A.M. and Price, D. (2011) 'The final frontier: The UK's new coalition government turns the English National Health Service over to the global health care market', *Health Sociology Review*, 20(3): 294–305.

Portus, J., Lopera, J.A., Baron, J., Diez, J.L., Falomir, M., Finaldi, G., Glendinning, N., Marques, M.B.M., Sanchez, A.E.P., Gomez, L.R. and Maroto, P.S. (2004) *The Spanish Portrait: From El Greco to Picasso*, Museo Nacional Del Prado, London: Scala Publishers.

Powell, W. and DiMaggio, P. (1991) (eds) *The New Institutionalism in Organizational Analysis*, University of Chicago Press, Chicago.

Pringle, R. (1998) *Sex and Medicine: Gender, Power and Authority in the Medical Profession*. Cambridge: Cambridge University Press.

Pulver, L., Haswell, M., Ring, I., Waldon, Clark, W., Whetung, V., Kinnon, D., Graham, C., Chino, M., Lavalley, J. and Sadana, R. (2010) *Indigenous Health? Australia, Canada, Aotearoa New Zealand and the United States: Laying Claim to a Future that Embraces Health for Us All*, World Health Report: Background Paper 33, Geneva: World Health Organization.

Ransome, W. and Sampford, C.J. (2012) 'Building an ethical and sustainable model for health professional recruitment', In S. Short and F. McDonald (eds) *Health Workforce Governance: Improved Access, Good Regulatory Practice, Safer Patients*, pp. 41–56, United Kingdom: Ashgate.

Reading, C. and Wein, F. (2009) *Health Inequalities and Social Determinants of Aboriginal Peoples' Health*, British Columbia: Canada National Collaborating Centre for Aboriginal Health, Prince George.

Rechel, B., Mladovsky, P., Devillé, W., Rijks, B., Petrova-Benedict, R. and McKee, M. (2011) 'Migration and health in the European Union: An introduction', In B. Rechel, P. Mladovsky, W. Devillé, B. Rijks, R. Petrova-Benedict and M. McKee (eds) *Migration and Health in the European Union*, pp. 3–16, Maidenhead: Open University Press and McGraw-Hill.

Rees, S., Rodley, G. and Stilwell, F. (eds) (1993) *Beyond the Market: Alternatives to Economic Rationalism*, Sydney: Pluto Press.

Reid, J.C. (1982) (ed.) *Body, Land and Spirit: Health and Healing in Aboriginal Society*, St Lucia, Qld: University of Queensland Press.

Reiger, K. (2011) ' "Knights or knaves"?: Public policy, professional power, and reforming maternity services', *Heath Care Women International*, 32(1): 2–22.

Reiger, K. and Morton, C. (2012) 'Standardizing or individualizing? A critical analysis of the "discursive imaginaries" shaping maternity care reform', *International Journal of Childbirth*, 2(3): 173–86.

Reiss, H.S. (ed.) (1991) *Kant: Political Writings*, Cambridge Texts in the History of Political Thought, Cambridge University Press, Cambridge.

Reynolds, H. (2005) *Nowhere People*, Melbourne: Penguin.

Reynolds, H. (1996) *Aboriginal Sovereignty: Reflections on Race, State and Nation*, Sydney: Allen & Unwin.

Reynolds, H. (1981) *The Other Side of the Frontier: An Interpretation of the Aboriginal Response to the Invasion and Settlement of Australia*, Townsville: History Department, James Cook University.

Rifkin, S.B. (2003) 'A framework linking community empowerment and health equity: It is a matter of choice', *Journal of Population Health and Nutrition*, 21(3): 168–80.

Riis, J. (1890) *How the Other Half Lives: Studies Among the Tenements of New York*, New York: Charles Scribner's Sons. Accessed at: www.bartleby.com/208/10.html, 4 September 2014.

Ritzer, G. (ed.) (2007) *The Blackwell Encyclopedia of Sociology*, Oxford: Blackwell.

Robinson, W.I. (2012) 'Global capitalism theory and the emergence of transnational elites', *Critical Sociology*, 38(3): 349–63.

Robson, B., Purdie, G. and Cormack, D. (2010) *Unequal Impact II: Māori and Non-Māori Cancer Statistics by Deprivation and Rural–Urban Status, 2002–2006*, Wellington: NZ Ministry of Health.

Rogers, L. (2010) 'Sexing the brain: The science and pseudoscience of sex differences', *The Kaioshung Journal of Medical Sciences*, 26(6): S4–9.

Rogers, L. (2000) *Sexing the Brain*, London: Phoenix.

Rohde, J., Cousens, S., Chopra, M., Tangcharoensathien, V., Black, R., Bhutta, Z.A. and Lawn, J.E. (2008) 'Thirty years after Alma-Ata: Has primary health care worked in countries?' *Lancet*, 372(9642): 950–61.

Rosen, G. (1963) 'The hospital: Historical sociology of a community institution', In E. Freidson (ed.) *The Hospital in Modern Society*, pp. 1–36, New York: Free Press of Glencoe.

Roth, L.M. and Henley, M.M. (2012) 'Unequal motherhood: Racial-ethnic and socioeconomic disparities in cesarean sections in the United States', *Social Problems*, 59(2): 207–27.

Rowse, T. (2009) 'The ontological politics of "closing the gaps" ', *Journal of Cultural Economy*, 2(1–2): 33–48.

Roy, A. (2014) 'Senate republicans develop the most credible plan yet to repeal and replace Obamacare', *Forbes*, 27 January 2014. Accessed at: www.forbes.com/sites/theapothecary/2014/01/27/senate-republicans-develop-the-most-credible-plan-yet-to-repeal-and-replace-obamacare/, 23 February 2014.

Russell, C. and Schofield, T. (1986) *Where it Hurts: An Introduction to Sociology for Health Workers*, Sydney: Allen & Unwin.

Ryan, L. (2012) *Tasmanian Aborigines: A History Since 1803*, Sydney: Allen & Unwin.

Rylko-Baurer, B. and Farmer, F. (2002) 'Managed care or managed inequality? A call for critiques of market-based medicine', *Medical Anthropology Quarterly*, 16(4): 476–502.

Saenz, L. (1985) 'Health changes during a decade: The Costa Rican case', In S.B. Halstead, J.A. Walsh and K.S. Warren (eds) *Good Health at Low Cost*, pp. 139–45, New York: Rockefeller Foundation.

Said, E. (1978) *Orientalism*, London: Routledge & Kegan Paul.

Sanders, T. and Harrison, S. (2008) 'Professional legitimacy claims in the multidisciplinary workplace: The case of heart failure care', *Sociology of Health and Illness*, 30(2): 289–308.

Savage, M., Devine, F., Cunningham, N., Taylor, M., Li, Y., Hjellbrekke, J., Le Roux, B., Friedman, S. and Miles, A. (2013) 'A new model of social class? Findings from the BBC's Great British Class Survey Experiment', *Sociology*, 47(2): 219–50.

Schmitt, C. (2008) *The Leviathan in the State Theory of Thomas Hobbes: Meaning and Failure of a Political Symbol*, Chicago: University of Chicago Press.

Schofield, T. (2014) 'Workplace health', In J. Germov (ed.) *Second Opinion: An Introduction to Health Sociology*, 5th edn, pp. 103–21, Melbourne: Oxford University Press.

Schofield, T. (2012a) 'Men's health and wellbeing', In E. Kuhlmann and E. Annandale (eds) *The Palgrave Handbook of Gender and Healthcare*, pp. 273–89, Houndmills, Basingstoke: Palgrave Macmillan.

Schofield, T. (2012b) 'The global health workforce "crisis" and inequities in health care access: Advancing a gender and organisations approach to policy, research and practice', In S.D. Short and F. McDonald (eds) *Health Workforce Governance: Improved Access, Good Regulatory Practice, Safer Patients*, pp. 57–76, Farnham: Ashgate.

Schofield, T. (2009) 'Gendered organisational dynamics: The elephant in the room for Australian allied health workforce policy and planning?' *Journal of Sociology*, 45(4): 383–400.

Schofield, T. (2007) 'Health inequity and its social determinants: A sociological commentary', *Health Sociology Review*, 16(2): 105–14.

Schofield, T. (2004) *Boutique Health? Gender and Equity in Health Policy*, Australian Health Policy Institute Commissioned Paper Series 2004/08, Sydney: The University of Sydney.

Schofield, T. (1990) 'Living with disability', In J. Reid, J. and P. Trompf, P. (eds) *The Health of Immigrant Australia*, pp. 288–311, Sydney and New York: Harcourt Brace Jovanovich.

Schofield, T., Connell, R.W., Walker, T. and Wood, J. (2000) 'Understanding men's health and illness: A gender-relations approach to policy, research, and practice', *Journal of American College Health*, 48(6): 247–56.

Schofield, T. and Goodwin, S. (2005) 'Gender politics and public policy making: Prospects for advancing gender equality', *Policy and Society*, 24(4): 25–44.

Schofield, T., Reeve, B. and McCallum, R. (2014) 'Australian workplace health and safety regulatory approaches to prosecution: Hegemonising compliance', *Journal of Industrial Relations*, published online 17 January.

Schulpen, T.W. (1996) 'Migration and child health: The Dutch experience', *European Journal of Pediatatrics*, 155(5): 351–6.

Schumpeter, J.A. (1943/1987) *Capitalism, Socialism, and Democracy*, London: Allen & Unwin.

Scott, J.T. (2012) *The Major Political Writings of Jean-Jacques Rousseau: The Two Discourses and the Social Contract*, translated and edited by J.T. Scott, Chicago and London: University of Chicago Press.

Scott, K. (2010) *That Deadman Dance*, Sydney: Picador.

Sebastian, T. and Donelly, M. (2013) 'Policy influences affecting the food practices of Indigenous Australians since colonisation', *Australian Aboriginal Studies: Journal of the Australian Institute of Aboriginal and Torres Strait Islander Studies*, 2: 59–75.

Senate Standing Committee on Legal and Constitutional Affairs (2006) *Unfinished Business: Indigenous Stolen Wages*, Canberra: Commonwealth of Australia.

Shakespeare T. (2006) *Disability Rights and Wrongs*, Abingdon, UK: Routledge.

Shapiro, I. (ed.) (2003) *Two Treatises of Government: And a Letter Concerning Toleration/John Locke*, New Haven, Connecticut: Yale University Press.

Shleifer, A. and Vishny, R.W. (1994) 'Politicians and firms', *The Quarterly Journal of Economics*, 109(4): 995–1025.

Singh, G.K. and Siahpush, M. (2006) 'Widening socioeconomic inequalities in US life expectancy, 1980–2000', *International Journal of Epidemiology*, 35(4): 969–79.

Singh, M. & de Looper, M. (2002) 'Australian health inequalities: 1 Birthplace', *Bulletin* no. 2. AIHW Catalogue No. AUS 27. Canberra: Australian Institute of Health and Welfare. Accessed at: www.aihw.gov.au/WorkArea/DownloadAsset.aspx?id=6442453153, 4 February 2014.

Sitas, F., Parkin, M., Chirenje, M., Stein, L., Abratt, R. and Wabinga, H. (2008) 'Part 2: Cancer in Indigenous Africans: Causes and controls', *Lancet*, 9: 786–95.

Siverbo, S. (2004) 'The purchaser–provider split in principle and practice: Experiences from Sweden', *Financial Accountability & Management*, 20(4): 401–20. doi: 10.1111/j.1468-0408.2004.00201.x.

Slack, P. (1988) 'Responses to plague in early modern Europe: The implications of public health', *Social Research*, 55(3): 433–53.

Smedley, A. and Smedley, B.D. (2005) 'Race as biology is fiction, racism as a social problem is real: Anthropological and historical perspectives on the social construction of race', *American Psychologist*, 60(1): 16–26.

Smedley, B.D., Stith, A.Y. and Nelson, A.R. (2003) *Unequal Treatment: Confronting Racial and Ethnic Disparities in Health Care*, Washington, DC: National Academies Press.

Smith, A. (1763) *Lectures On Jurisprudence*, In R.L. Meek, D.D. Raphael and P.G. Stein (eds) (1978), New York: Clarendon Press and Oxfordshire: Oxford University Press.

Smith, L.T. (2012) *Decolonizing Methodologies: Research and Indigenous Peoples*, London: Zed Books.

Solonec, C. (2013) 'Proper mixed-up: Miscegenation among Aboriginal Australians', *Australian Aboriginal Studies: Journal of the Australian Institute of Aboriginal and Torres Strait Islander Studies*, 2: 76–85.

Starfield, B. (2011) 'The hidden inequity in health care', *International Journal of Equity Health*, 10: 15.

Starfield, B., Shi, L. and Macinko, J. (2005). 'Contribution of primary care to health systems and health', *The Millbank Quarterly*, 83(3): 457–502.

Starr, P. (1982). *The Social Transformation of American Medicine: The Rise of a Sovereign Profession and the Making of a Vast Industry*, New York: Basic Books.

Statistics Canada (2005) *Canadian Community Health Survey*. Accessed at: http://www5.statcan.gc.ca/cansim/a05, 8 February 2014.

Statistics New Zealand (2013) *New Zealand Periodic Lifetables: 2010–12*. Accessed at: www.stats.govt.nz, 26 April 2014.

Steele, C., Cardinez, C., Richardson, L., Tom-Orme, L. and Shaw, K. (2008) 'Surveillance for health behaviours of American Indians and Alaska natives: Findings from the behavioural risk factor surveillance system: 2000–2006', *Supplement to Cancer*, 113(5): 1131–41.

Stiglitz, J.E. (2008) 'Is there a post-Washington-consensus consensus?' In N. Serra and J.E. Stiglitz (eds) *The Washington Consensus Reconsidered: Towards a New Global Governance*, New York: Oxford University Press.

Stiglitz, J.E. (2002) *Globalization and Its Discontents*, New York: Norton.

Stiglitz, J.E. (2000) 'Capital market liberalization, economic growth and instability', *World Development*, 28(6): 1075–86.

Stiglitz, J.E. and Lin-Yifu (2014) *The Industrial Policy Revolution I: The Role of Government Beyond Ideology*, International Economic Association Series, Houndmills: Palgrave Macmillan.

Stilwell, F. and Jordan, K. (2007) *Who Gets What? Analysing Economic Inequality in Australia*, Cambridge: Cambridge University Press.

Stoler, A. (1995) *Race and the Education of Desire: Foucault's History of Sexuality and the Colonial Order of Things*, Durham: Duke University Press.

Stoner, L., Stoner, K. and Fryer, S. (2012) 'Preventing a cardiovascular disease epidemic among Indigenous populations through lifestyle changes', *International Journal of Preventative Medicine*, 3(4): 230–40.

Straus, S. (2013) 'Africa is becoming more peaceful, despite the war in Mali', *The Guardian*. Accessed at: www.guardian.co.uk/world/2013/jan/30/africa-peaceful-mali-war, 9 March 2013.

Streefland, P. (2005) 'Public health care under pressure in sub-Saharan Africa', *Health Policy*, 71(3): 375–82.

Stringer, C. (2012) *Lone Survivors: How We Come To Be the Only Humans on Earth*, New York: Henry Holt & Company.

Sutherland, K. (ed.) (2008) *An Inquiry into the Nature and Causes of the Wealth of Nations: A Selected Edition/Adam Smith*, Oxford: Oxford University Press.

Swamy, A. (2011) 'Land and law in colonial India', In D. Ma and J. Luiten Van Zanden (eds) *Long-term Economic Change in Eurasian Perspective*, Stanford: Stanford University Press.

Taylor, A. (2013) '26 years of growth: Shanghai then and now', *The Atlantic*, 7 August, Accessed at: http://www.theatlantic.com/infocus/2013/08/26-years-of-growth-shanghai-then-and-now/100569/, 8 July 2014.

Thatcher, M. (1987) Interview with Douglas Keay for *Woman's Own*, 23 September, London. Accessed at: www.margaretthatcher.org/document/106689, 20 April 2013.

Thompson, E.P. (1993) *Customs in Common*, London: Penguin.

Thompson, E.P. (1980) *The Making of the English Working Class*, Harmondsworth: Penguin.

Thomson, S., Osborn, R., Squires, D. and Jun, M. (eds) (2013) *International Profiles of HealthCare Systems*. The Commonwealth Fund. Accessed at: www.commonwealthfund.org/~/media/Files/Publications/Fund%20Report/2013/Nov/1717_Thomson_intl_profiles_hlt_care_sys_2013_v2.pdf, 27 January 2014.

Trowler, P. (1984) *Topics in Sociology*, Slough: University Tutorial Press.

Tudor-Hart, J.T. (1971) 'The Inverse Care Law', *Lancet*, i: 405–12.

Tully, J. (2012) 'Rethinking human rights and Enlightenment: A view from the twenty-first century', In K.E. Tunstall (ed.) *Self-Evident Truths?: Human Rights and the Enlightenment*, New York: Bloomsburry, pp. 3–34.

Tynkkynen, L.K., Keskimäki, I and Lehto, J. (2013) 'Purchaser–provider splits in health care: The case of Finland', *Health Policy*, 111(3): 221–5.

United Health Foundation (2011) *America's health rankings: A call to action for individuals and their communities*. Accessed at: http://cdnfiles.americashealthrankings.org/SiteFiles/Reports/AHR%202011edition.pdf, 27 April 2013.

United Nations (UN) (2013) *Human Development Report*. Accessed at: http://hdr.undp.org/en/2013-report, 23 June 2014.

UN (2010) *The World's Women: Trends and Statistics*, Department of Economic and Social Affairs, New York. Accessed at: http://unstats.un.org/unsd/demographic/products/Worldswomen/WW2010pub.htm, 5 September 2014.

United Nations Children's Fund (UNICEF) (2014) *UNICEF Data: Monitoring the Situation of Children and Women: Maternal Mortality*. Accessed at: http://data.unicef.org/maternal-health/maternal-mortality.

UNICEF (2013) *Nigeria*. Accessed at: www.unicef.org/nigeria/children_1926.html, 26 July 2013.

United Nations Development Programme (UNDP) (2012) 'Rickshaw drivers prosper with new services', *Southern Innovator: Transforming the Global South*. Accessed at: http://www.southerninnovator.org/index.php/innovation/59, 9 September 2013.

United Nations Statistics Division (2012) 'Social indicators: Work'. Accessed at: http://unstats.un.org/unsd/demographic/products/socind/, 17 September 2013.

United States Centers for Disease Control and Prevention (2013) *Health Disparities and Inequalities Report: US 2013*. Accessed at: www.cdc.gov/mmwr/pdf/other/su6203.pdf, 26 April 2014.

United States Department of Health and Human Services (US DHHS) (2013) *America's Children: Key National Indicators of Well-Being: 2013*. Accessed at: www.childstats.gov/americaschildren, 26 April 2014.

US DHHS (2011) *Health, United States, 2010: With Special Feature on Death and Dying*. Accessed at: www.cdc.gov/nchs/data/hus/hus10.pdf, 17 January 2014.

United States Federal Bureau of Prisons (2009) *Quick Facts About the Bureau of Prisons*. Accessed at: www.bop.gov/news/quick.jsp, 4 September 2014.

United States Substance Abuse and Mental Health Services Administration, Office of Applied Studies (2010) *The NSDUH Report: Substance Use among American Indian or Alaska Native Adults*. Accessed at: www.samsha.org, 26 April 2014.

Van Krieken, R., Habibis, D., Hutchins, B., Martin, G. and Maton, K. (eds) (2014) *Sociology*, 5th edn, Frenchs Forest, NSW: Pearson.

Vargas, J.C. (2005). *Nicaraguans in Costa Rica and the United States: Data from Ethnic Surveys*, Los Angeles: California Centre for Population Research.

Vearey, J. (2013) 'Migrant health and inequalities: Reflections on the experiences of Latin American migrants in London', In T. Bastia (ed.) *Migration and Inequality*, pp. 187–207, London: Routledge.

Wagstaff, A. and van Doorslaer, E. (2003) 'Catastrophe and impoverishment in paying for health care: With applications to Vietnam 1993–1998', *Health Economics*, 12(11): 921–33.

Wajcman, J. (1999) *Managing Like a Man: Women and Men in Corporate Management*, Cambridge: Polity Press and Sydney: Allen & Unwin.

Wakim, J. (2006) 'A police disservice to paint race relations with broad-brush labels', *The Sydney Morning Herald*, 1 February 2006.

Walby, S. (1986) *Patriarchy at Work*, Cambridge: Polity Press.

Waldby, C. and Mitchell, R. (2006) *Tissue Economies: Blood, Organs, and Cell Lines in Late Capitalism*, Durham, NC: Duke University Press.

Waldron, I. (1967) 'Why do women live longer than men?', *Social Science & Medicine*, 10 (7–8): 349–62.

Walker, L., Butland, D. and Connell, R.W. (2000) 'Boys on the road: Masculinities, car culture, and road safety education', *Journal of Men's Studies*, 8(2): 153–69.

Walters, D. and Nichols, T. (2007) *Worker Representation and Workplace Health and Safety*, Basingstoke: Palgrave Macmillan.

Waring, M. (1988) *Counting for Nothing: What Men Value and What Women are Worth*, Sydney: Allen & Unwin.

Weatherburn, D. (2014) *Arresting Incarceration: Pathways out of Indigenous Imprisonment*, Canberra: Aboriginal Studies Press.

Weber, M. (1930/1974) *The Protestant Ethic and the Spirit of Capitalism*, London: Unwin University Books.

Weller, M. and Nobbs, K. (eds) (2010) *Political Participation of Minorities: A Commentary on International Standards and Practice*, New York: Oxford University Press.

Wester, S.R., Vogel, D.L., Pressly, P.K. and Heesacker, M. (2002) 'Sex differences in emotion: A critical review of the literature and implications for counselling psychology', *The Counselling Psychologist*, 30(4): 630–52.

White, R. (2008) 'Class analysis and the crime problem', In T. Anthony and C. Cuneen (eds) *The Critical Criminology Companion*, pp. 30–42, Leichhardt, NSW: Hawkins Press.

Whiteside, H. (2011) 'Unhealthy policy: The political economy of Canadian public-private partnership hospitals', *Health Sociology Review*, 20(3): 258–68.

Whittaker, W. (2008), 'Pleasure and pain: Medical travel in Asia', *Global Public Health*, 3(3): 271–90.

Wicks, D. (1998) *Nurses and Doctors at Work: Rethinking Professional Barriers*, Buckingham: Open University Press.

Wiggins, C., Espey, D., Wingo, P., Kaur, J., Wilson, R., Swan, J., Miller, B., Jim, M., Kelly, J. and Lanier, A. (2008) 'Cancer among American Indians and Alaska natives in the United States: 1999–2004', *Supplement to Cancer*, 113(5): 1142–52.

Wilenski, P. (1987) *Public Power and Public Administration*, Sydney: Hale & Iremonger.

Wilkinson, R. and Marmot, M. (eds) (2003) *Social Determinants of Health: The Solid Facts*, 2nd edn, Copenhagen: World Health Organization, Regional Office for Europe.

Williams, D. (ed.) (1999) *The Enlightenment*, Cambridge: Cambridge University Press.

Williams, D.R. and Jackson, P.B. (2005) 'Social sources of racial disparities in health', *Health Affairs*, 24(2): 325–34.

Williams, D.R. and Mohammed, S.A. (2013) 'Racism and health II: A needed research agenda for effective interventions', *American Behavioral Scientist*, 57(8): 1200–26.

Williams, L. and Lawlis, T. (2014) 'Jostling for position: A sociology of allied health', In J. Germov (ed.) *Second Opinion: An Introduction to Health Sociology*, pp. 439–63, Melbourne: Oxford University Press.

Williams, R. (1976) *Keywords: A Vocabulary of Culture and Society*, Glasgow: Fontana/Croom Helm.

Willis, E. (2006). 'Introduction: Taking stock of medical dominance', *Health Sociology Review*, 15: 421–31.

Willis, E. (1989) *Medical Dominance: The Division of Labour in Australian Health Care*, revised edn, Sydney: Allen & Unwin.

Willis, E. (1983) *Medical Dominance: The Division of Labour in Australian Health Care*, Sydney: Allen & Unwin.

Willis, P. with Jones, S., Canaan, J. and Hurd, G. (1990) *Common Culture: Symbolic Work at Play in the Everyday Cultures of the Young*, Milton Keynes, UK: Open University Press.

Willmot, E. (1988) *Pemulwuy: The Rainbow Warrior*, Sydney: Bantam.

Wolf, E.R. (1982) *Europe and the People Without History*, Berkeley and Los Angeles: University of California Press.

Wood, C.S. (1979) *Human Sickness and Health: A Biocultural View*, Palo Alto, California: Mayfield Publishing.

Woodward, C.V. (2002) *The Strange Career of Jim Crow: A Commemorative Edition*, New York: Oxford University Press.

World Bank (2014a) *1.5 World Development Indicators. World View: Women in Development.* Accessed at: http://wdi.worldbank.org/table/1.5, 23 August 2014.

World Bank (2014b) *2.2 World Development Indicators: Labor Force Structure.* Accessed at: http://wdi.worldbank.org/table/2.2, 12 June 2014.

World Bank (2014c) *2.21 World Development Indicators: Mortality.* Accessed at http://wdi. worldbank.org/table/2.21, 12 June 2014.

World Bank (2014d) *2.3 World Development Indicators. People: Employment by Sector.* Accessed at: http://wdi.worldbank.org/table/2.3, 23 August 2014.

World Bank (2014e) *Data By Topic: Poverty.* Accessed at: http://data.worldbank.org/topic/poverty, 2 September 2014.

World Bank (2014f) 'GDP ranking: Gross domestic product 2012', *World Development Indicators,* Accessed at: http://data.worldbank.org/data-catalog/GDP-ranking-table, 30 April 2014.

World Bank (2013) *Life Expectancy at Birth,* Accessed at: http://data.worldbank.org/indicator/SP.DYN.LE00.IN, 24 June 2014.

World Bank (2012) *De-Fragmenting Africa: Deepening Regional Trade Integration in Goods and Services,* Washington D.C.: World Bank. Accessed at: http://documents.worldbank.org/curated/en/2012/01/16252822/de-fragmenting-africa-deepening-regional-trade-integration-goods-services, 26 July 2013.

World Bank (2008) *Health Workers Needed: Poor Left Without Care in Africa's Rural Areas.* Accessed at: http://go.worldbank.org/IUY3J2M0A0, 11 February 2014.

World Health Organization (WHO) (2014a) *Trends in Maternal Mortality: 1990 to 2013: Estimates by WHO, UNICEF, UNFPA, The World Bank and the United Nations Population Division.*

WHO (2014b) *World Health Statistics.* Accessed at: http://www.who.int/gho/publications/world_health_statistics/2014/en/, 3 September 2014.

WHO (2013a) *Global Tuberculosis Report,* Geneva: WHO Accessed at: www.who.int/tb/publications/global_report/en/, 21 June 2014.

WHO (2013b) *Global Update on HIV Treatment 2013: Results, Impact and Opportunities,* WHO Report in Partnership with UNICEF and UNAIDS, Geneva: WHO.

WHO (2013c) *Life Expectancy: Life Expectancy Data by Country,* Global Health Observatory Data Repository. Accessed at: http://apps.who.int/gho/data/node.main.688, 26 July 2013.

WHO (2013d) *Preterm Birth. Fact Sheet No. 363.* Accessed at www.who.int/mediacentre/factsheets/fs363/en/, 3 March 2014.

WHO (2013e) *Overweight/Obesity: Overweight (body mass index >25) Data by Country,* Global Health Observatory Data Repository. Accessed at: http://apps.who.int/gho/data/node.main. A897?lang=en, 26 July 2013.

WHO (2013f) *Road Traffic Injuries. Fact Sheet No. 358.* Accessed at: http://www.who.int/medicentre/factshetts/fs358/en/, 2 September 2014.

WHO (2010a) *Action on the Social Determinants of Health: Learning From Previous Experiences.* Accessed at: www.who.int/social_determinants/corner/en/, 25 June 2014.

WHO (2010b) *Injuries and Violence: The Facts.* Accessed at: www.who.int/violence_injury_prevention/key_facts/en/, 2 September 2014.

WHO (2010c) *10 Facts on Gender and Tobacco*. Accessed at: www.who.int/features/factfiles/gender_tobacco/en/, 2 September 2014.

WHO (2009a) *Gender Disparities in Mental Health*. Accessed at: www.who.int/mental_health/media/en/242.pdf, 2 September 2014.

WHO (2009b) *Global Health Risks: Mortality and Burden of Disease Attributable to Selected Major Risks*. Accessed at: www.who.int/healthinfo/global_burden_disease/GlobalHealthRisks_report_full.pdf, 25 March 2013.

WHO (2008) *The World Health Report 2008: Primary Health Care Now More Than Ever*, Geneva: WHO.

WHO (2007) *Everybody's Business: Strengthening Health Systems to Improve Health Outcomes*, Geneva: WHO.

WHO (2006) *The World Health Report: Working Together for Health*, Geneva: WHO. Accessed at: http://apps.who.int/iris/bitstream/10665/43471/1/9241594241_eng.pdf?ua=1, 24 June 2014.

WHO (2005a) *Gender, Health and Alcohol Use*. Accessed at: www.who.int/gender/documents/Alcoholfinal.pdf, 4 September 2014.

WHO (2005b) *Multi-country Study on Women's Health and Domestic Violence Against Women: Initial Results on Prevalence, Health Outcomes and Women's Responses*, Geneva: WHO.

WHO (2001) *WHO's Contribution to the World Conference Against Racism, Racial Discrimination, Xenophobia and Related Intolerance: Health and Freedom From Discrimination*, Health and Human Rights Publication Series, Issue 2.

WHO (1990) *The Concepts and Principles of Equity in Health*, Copenhagen: WHO Regional Office for Europe, EUR/ICP/RPD 414.

WHO (1948) *Preamble to the Constitution of the World Health Organization as Adopted by the International Health Conference, New York, 19–22 June, 1946; signed on 22 July 1946 by the representatives of 61 States (Official Records of the World Health Organization, no. 2, p. 100) and entered into force on 7 April 1948*. Accessed at: www.who.int/governance/eb/constitution/en, 19 March 2013.

WHO and UNICEF (2013) *Water, Sanitation and Hygiene*, Geneva. Accessed at: www.unicef.org/wash/index_statistics.html, 21 June 2014.

World Heart Federation (2014) 'Indigenous health/rheumatic heart disease', *Proceedings of the World Congress on Cardiology*, Melbourne, Australia. Accessed at: www.world-heart-federation.org/, 1 May 2014.

Wright, E.O. (ed.) (2005) *Approaches to Class Analysis*, Cambridge: Cambridge University Press.

Xu, K., Evans, D.B., Carrin G., Aguilar-Rivera, A.M., Musgrove P. and Evans T. (2007) 'Protecting households from catastrophic health spending', *Health Affairs*, 26: 972–83.

Yeatman, A. (1990) *Bureaucrats, Technocrats, Femocrats: Essays on the Contemporary Australian State*, Sydney: Allen & Unwin.

Yoon, T.H., Lee, S.Y., Kim, C.W., Kim, S.Y., Jeong, B.G. and Park, H.K. (2011) 'Inequalities in medical care utilization by South Korean cancer patients according to income: A retrospective cohort study', *International Journal of Health Services*, 41(1): 51–66.

Yuan, L. (2012) 'Older Miao People and Rural Health Policy in China', PhD thesis, University of Sydney.

Zola, E. (1885/1994) *Germinal*, translated by H. Ellis, New York: Vintage Books, Random House.

Index